P9-BZH-108

You Go Girl

BUT ONLY WHEN YOU WANT TO!

This book was made possible by an unrestricted educational grant from

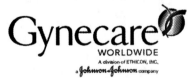

Gynecare
WORLDWIDE
A division of ETHICON, INC,
a *Johnson-Johnson* company

All proceeds from the sale of this book will go to educational initiatives,
community-based programs, and the further advancement
of pelvic health research.

You Go Girl

BUT ONLY WHEN YOU WANT TO!

KEY TIPS, TOPICS AND EXERCISES FOR
A HEALTHY, PASSIONATE, EXCITED YOU

MISSY D. LAVENDER

DOROTHY B. SMITH

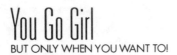

You Go Girl
BUT ONLY WHEN YOU WANT TO!

by Missy D. Lavender and Dorothy B. Smith

Copyright © 2007
Women's Health Foundation. All rights reserved.
Published by Women's Health Foundation, Chicago Illinois.

No part of this publication may be reproduced, stored in a retrieval system, or trans-
mitted in any form or by any means, electronic, mechanical, photocopying, recording,
scanning, or otherwise, except as permitted under Section 107 or 108 of the 1976
United States Copyright Act, without the prior written permission of the Publisher.
Requests to the Publisher for permission should be addressed to Missy Lavender,
Women's Health Foundation, 632 W. Deming Place, Chicago, IL 60618.

Limit of Liability/Disclaimer of Warranty: While the publisher and author have used
their best efforts in preparing this book, they make no representations or warranties
with respect to the accuracy or completeness of the contents of this book and specifically disclaim any implied warranties of merchantability or fitness for a particular
purpose. No warranty may be created or extended by sales representatives or written
sales materials. The advice and strategies contained herein may not be suitable for
your situation. You should consult with a professional where appropriate. Neither
the publisher nor author shall be liable for any loss of profit or any other commercial
damages, including but not limited to special, incidental, consequential, or other
damages.

Editor: Training Systems Inc., www.trainingsys.com
Editor: Merle Levenstein
Copyeditor: Molly Kirk, www.womenshealthfoundation.org
Interior design: Toolbox Creative, www.ToolboxCreative.com
Cover Design: Phillip Newswanger, www.mododesigngroup.com

Library of Congress Cataloguing-in-Publications Data
Library of Congress Control Number: 2007931538
Missy D. Lavender and Dorothy B. Smith
You Go Girl...but Only When You Want To!: Key Tips, Topics And Exercises For
A Healthy, Passionate, Excited You
ISBN: 978-0-9796876-0-0
Library of Congress subject headings:
1. Women's Health
2007931538
2007

*This Book contains general information that may not be applicable to your
specific situation. It should not be used as a substitute for the advice of a
doctor or medical professional.*

DEDICATION

In Memory of my grandmother, Elma Morton Fallon,
who loved and inspired me

Acknowledgements

It has been an honor to be a part of the creation of this book. I am pleased to have had the opportunity through it to share some of the important principles, tips and topics I have learned in the past seven years. I drew from my own experiences first as a new mom with an out-of-control bladder, then as a patient and advocate and, finally, as one of the millions of perimenopausal woman wondering "what is happening to my body down there?" From speaking with thousands of women through the Total Control™ program, it is clear that women are sorely lacking in basic knowledge about bladder and pelvic health. We do not know about it, we do not honor it, and we certainly do not talk about anything until we have become a complete disaster. Our intent with this book is to be informative and seductive enough to get women back into their bodies by inspiring them to be interested, motivated and empowered.

I would like to thank my team at Women's Health Foundation, specifically Molly Kirk, Lauren Sylvester and Amelia Manderscheid, for their help and dedication to this project. It has been a learning opportunity for us all.

I would like to thank Dr. Linda Brubaker at Loyola University Medical Center for her warmth and compassion, for her support and encouragement from the first day we met. Her guidance and contacts in the field of urogynecology were incredibly helpful. I am honored to have worked with you and I think you are the absolute best.

Another big thank you goes to Kim Wilschek at Alberto-Culver's Women's Health Center for her editing and formatting help, her willingness to champion women's pelvic health and for her friendship and expertise.

I would like to express my gratitude to Michael Wax at DesChutes Medical for the opportunity to have this project in the first place and for his generosity with our organization. We look forward to future endeavors with you.

Dot Smith, thank you for having the initial idea for this publication and for your co-authorship. Your original book, "Bladder Control is No Accident," was so helpful to thousands of women and is the foundation for our work. Without you and Michael, our vision might not have been realized.

Thank you Dr. Roger Goldberg. Your book inspired me; your humor makes me laugh. I am honored to have you on our team. Thank you, too, for generously sharing your work with us and for collaborating with us on this book.

Thank you to Gynecare for your generous sponsorship and support throughout this project. Your commitment to our organization made this book a reality.

Abundant thanks to the entire Total Control™ team, especially Mary Drill, Judy Florendo and Maureen George. You have all been such wonderful leaders and spent endless hours focusing on women's pelvic fitness. I cannot thank you enough for your willingness to give of yourselves and your time, and for sharing my passion for bringing women "out of the water closet and into the gym!" We *are* changing the world, one pelvic floor at a time.

My deepest thanks to my son, Wiley, for your love, your cuddles in the early morning and for your snuggles at night. To my sweet daughter, Fallon, thank you for your spirit and energy and for your kisses and hugs as I come in the door every day. It makes it all worthwhile. I love you both and I know you will grow up knowing more than you imagined possible about the female pelvic floor. May it make your life and the lives of those you love stronger and healthier.

Lastly, but just as enthusiastically, thanks to my husband, Kim Redding, without whom none of this would be possible. Your love sustains me, completes me and helps keep everything in perspective. Thank you for your generosity from the beginning and for being interested and passionate. I know you are my greatest fan - and I, yours.

Table of Contents

INTRODUCTION
There IS Life Beyond Your Bladder

Ask yourself the following questions: Can you imagine not obsessing about going to the bathroom? How often you have to go? Where is the closest facility? Will you make it there without leaking? How much water should you drink (or not) before you go into your 1:00 p.m. meeting?

What if your bladder were "worry free?" What if you were able to laugh without leaking? What if you were able to get home and in the door before you had to go?

Millions of women spend a great deal of their time and emotional energy on just these questions. In addition to all the logistics of a life ruled by their bladders, women factor these bodily concerns into their sense of themselves. Do they feel sexy? Do they feel comfortable in their own skin? Can they put on an outfit and feel attractive? Or, are they totally disconnected from their own bodies, living life completely oblivious to pelvic health and fitness?

While there are other books on the market about topics like urinary incontinence and overactive bladder, we wanted to provide the essential and easily readable primer to help women understand why their pelvis is key to their viability as a person, a mother, a partner. By understanding what is inside the female pelvis and how each "part" works, you will become more informed about why you need to care for your body from the "inside out."

We will share key tips, topics and exercises that can change your life. We want you to know why what you eat and drink matters, why your pelvic floor exercises can make sex better for you and your partner, why how and when you go to the bathroom can contribute to problems with leaking or urge. Most importantly, we want you to learn that breaking bad habits can lead to Life Beyond Your Bladder.

In addition to improving your understanding about women's pelvic health, we will explain the Total Control™ program, which includes a series of exercises designed to strengthen the three supporting muscles of the pelvis. The Total Control™ program is a community-based fitness and educational program taught throughout the U.S. and Canada at hospitals and gyms. (For more information on Total Control™, go to www.totalcontroprogram.com. Look for details about ordering the Total Control™ DVD.)

We can help you live a fuller and more active life. Study our guidelines. Then "pay it forward." There are SO many women out there that need this information - your mother, sister, daughter and best friend. Share your knowledge with them and then let us know how everybody is doing by writing us at info@womenshealth-foundation.org.

> To all the women who have given up hope, not knowing what to do or who to talk with about their bodies…to those of you who have stopped doing the things you love to do…for every woman who is afraid to have sex or has lost interest in her body…this book is our gift to you. ~MDL

Ready yourself for your journey back to a healthy and passionate you. May this text teach and inspire you to be your best.

CHAPTER ONE
Bladder Control is No Accident

You do not have to be a control freak to want to have control over your bladder. Have you ever felt your bladder has more control over your lifestyle than you do? Does your bladder dictate when you have to go, where you have to go and how often you have to go? Consider the situations below and see if any sound familiar to you.

IS THIS YOU?

- Do you know every gas station or fast food stop between home and work?
- Do you deliberately stop drinking fluids so you won't leak as much?
- Are you insecure about exercising with a group for fear of leaking?
- Does coffee, tea, and/or diet soda "go right through" you?
- Have you recently had to go home and change your clothing after an accident?
- Does going to the bathroom interfere with your work?
- Do you look for a bathroom minutes after having just gone?
- Do you get up to go to the bathroom more than two times every night, sometimes not getting there in time?
- Are you the first in line at the restroom after the movie, school play, sports event?
- Do you need to regularly use a panty liner?
- Have you ever been embarrassed because you leaked urine during sexual activity?

∞ Do you leak when you stand? Laugh? Cough? Sneeze? Lift? Push?

If you have responded "yes" to any of the aforementioned situations, you are definitely not alone. If you are dealing with loss of bladder control, even if you are hesitant to accept the term "incontinence," you know the inconvenience and the pain of this problem. But relax. There are simple and effective treatment options available. Girl, it is time to come out of the water closet and greet your new life!

Loss of Bladder Control – Incidence & Prevalence

Bladder control, or the lack thereof, has a lot of official terminology and definitions. Urinary incontinence, also known as loss of bladder control, is when you lose urine uncontrollably. While considering it bothersome, many women will continue to tolerate this life-altering condition for years, too embarrassed to ask for help and unaware of available treatments. As one woman reported, "We go underground with our problem."

An estimated one in four adults with bladder control problems seeks professional help regarding this condition only after deciding it will not go away on its own. However life altering it may be, loss of bladder control is not life threatening. Many health care providers are quick to dismiss a woman's complaints, citing old age or a possible consequence of breast-feeding as a cause. A diaper or pad might be recommended as a quick fix. Nevertheless, looking beyond the inconvenience of damp undergarments, skirts and trousers, serious complications can arise from urinary leakage. The following facts are known about women with urinary incontinence:

Women suffering from urinary incontinence are more at risk for a variety of setbacks:

∞ for **falls** while hurrying to the toilet trying to prevent an "accident"

- for urinary tract **infections** and the associated complications
- for **skin** breakdown if urine remains on the skin in a pad or clothing
- to be admitted to a **long-term care** facility when other health problems exist
- **longer hospital** stays and more frequent admissions
- financial **costs** of buying pads and/or supplies
- for living with the possibility of **humiliating** "accidents"
- to feel stress about the location of toilets, even to the point of **restricting** travel or other activities

Medical literature and research have documented these consequences and discussed the significance of incontinence beyond quality-of life-issues:

- The **annual cost** to a person over the age of 65 with incontinence is estimated at **$3,565.** [1]
- **Incontinence supplies ranked** # 1 in 2001 projected revenue for medical products at $2.2 billion. [2]
- **Urinary incontinence impacts the quality of life more adversely than** hypertension, diabetes and just about **any other medical condition except perhaps clinical depression.** [3]

Even less discussed, but equally as debilitating, are the psychosocial, i.e. quality of life, issues that compound the bladder control problem. Many women report decreases in activity, social withdrawal and isolation, increases in anxiety and fear, even depression. The good news is that as the incontinence symptoms begin to improve, women report an improvement in their anxiety and over-all well being. Urinary leakage is not a "sometimes" symptom like a headache that occurs occasionally and then gets better. It can be, and usually is, a several-times-a-day challenging and frustrating symptom.

---

1   "Economic cost of urinary incontinence in 1995," Wagner TH & Hu T, Urology, 1998, 51(3): pgs 355-361.
2   *Medical Device & Diagnostic Industry,* Frost & Sullivan, December 2000: pgs 47-56.
3   "Pathophysiology of urge incontinence," Appell RA, *Contemporary Urology,* March 1999: pgs 1-6.

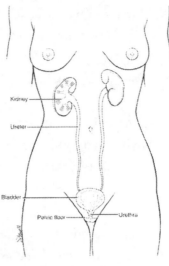

Kidney

Ureter

Bladder

Pelvic floor

Urethra

Bladder Basics

The Female Urinary Tract

THE BLADDER

The bladder is a fascinating organ in its design and functional capabilities. It has the responsibility of storing and emptying urine on command from the brain. It is an organ composed of muscle fibers that can stretch as it fills with urine. It has three openings: two for ureters (tubes) that drain urine into the bladder from the kidneys, one for the urethra (a tube that drains urine from the bladder to the outside of the body). At the base of the bladder, there are valves or sphincters which remain closed to keep urine in the bladder and open to let the bladder drain. When the bladder is full, the sphincters open and the bladder muscle contracts to force the urine out through the urethra.

THE URETHRA

Again, the urethra is the tube that drains urine from the bladder to the outside of the body. It is a pliable, elastic tubular organ that has several thick walls. The inner wall looks like folds with crevices. These crevices fill with secretions to make a better seal when the tube collapses for closure. The thickness, elasticity and moisture of the urethra are all important for a tight closure to keep urine from leaking.

In the female, the bladder is in front of the vagina, very close to the uterus. The urethra is short and exits in front of the vagina. The angle where the bladder joins the urethra is very important for urine control.

THE PELVIC FLOOR

Women have a series of muscles and ligaments in the pelvic floor which support the bladder, urethra and the other pelvic organs. These muscles are affected by strengthening exercises, estrogen levels and physical stress from childbirth, surgery and/or obesity.

HOW IT ALL WORKS

The kidneys make urine all the time. A trickle of urine is constantly passing to the bladder down the ureters (the tubes from the kidneys to the bladder). The amount of urine depends on how much you drink, eat and sweat. The bladder is made of muscle and expands like a balloon as it fills with urine. The outlet for urine (the urethra) is normally kept closed. This is helped by the muscles beneath the bladder that sweep around the urethra (the urethral sphincter and the pelvic floor muscles). When a certain amount of urine is in the bladder, you become aware that the bladder is getting full. When you go to the toilet to pass urine, the bladder muscle contracts (squeezes), and the urethra and pelvic floor muscles relax. Complex nerve messages are sent between the brain, the bladder and the pelvic floor muscles. You are, therefore, aware when your bladder is full. You instinctively contract or relax the right muscles at the right time.

Bladder control is a wondrous process when all is well. Because so many parts of the body are involved (the brain, spinal cord, branch nerves, blood vessels, bladder, urethra, hormones and pelvic muscles), there are numerous opportunities for some part or parts to work incorrectly.

Who Has This Problem?

Who, besides you, has this problem? Here are some real life examples. See if they sound familiar to you.

ANN

Ann is a 34 year-old homemaker and mother of three young children. Her youngest child is nine months old. After the birth of her third child, Ann leaked urine when she laughed, coughed, picked up her infant and even when she had sexual intercourse with her husband. She was very embarrassed and did not know where to turn for help. She started wearing menstrual pads, but they were not adequate enough to keep urine from spilling onto her clothing. Ann's doctor never discussed the common problem with her and she was too mortified to mention it. She thought she would have to live with the discomfort forever.

ANGIE

Angie is a 23-year-old competitive swimmer. She is single and very athletic. She works out with weights in the gym, swims, and jogs. For several years, Angie experienced urinary frequency and eventually began getting up to go to the bathroom four to five times a night. During the day, she even cut back on her fluid intake during exercise (self-dehydration) in an attempt to reduce her urinary frequency and leakage.

FRAN

Fran, age 83, lives in a retirement village. Several years ago, she began losing control of her bladder at night. Fran had been to several physicians and tried medications, but the medications made her dizzy causing her to fall and break her hip. They were discontinued. Now her caregiver awakes Fran every night at midnight to help her to the bathroom. Yet sometimes she still leaks, wetting her clothing and the bed. She has not had a full night's rest in months. Fran wears pads made for incontinence, but the smell of urine is ever present.

You might have a horror story of your own; you might know about the suffering of loved ones. Anne, Angie and Fran were successfully treated because they chose to be proactive, to seek help. The lesson is you can take positive action and regain your life.

We have reviewed basic bladder anatomy and physiology. Now let us discuss various kinds of bladder control problems and possible solutions.

CHAPTER TWO

Risks of Developing an "Out of Control Bladder"

According to the International Continence Society, the unexpected loss of urine that is considered "bothersome" is called urinary incontinence. While few women we have talked with will admit to being "incontinent," heads nod definitively "yes" when talking to a room of women about that "gotta go, gotta go" feeling. Doing jumping jacks and staying dry seems unimaginable. If properly surveyed, many women would, in fact, be considered incontinent.

While both men and women may develop bladder control problems, women have more risk factors simply by virtue of their anatomy and their giving birth. In fact, estimates range from 10-20% of all adult women struggle with bladder control issues.

WHO IS AT RISK

Stress Incontinence	Urge Incontinence
Women with children	Women with irritable bladder conditions such as interstitial cystitis
Women who do high impact exercise	Women with Overactive Bladder (OAB)
Women after menopause	Women with repeated sexual dysfunction and/or chronic pelvic pain
Women with a chronic cough	Women with chronic urinary tract infections ("UTI")
Women who are overweight	Women with diabetes or who are on prescription medications for heart disease or hypertension
Women who chronically strain to have a bowel movement	Women who have had pelvic surgery or a hysterectomy

Risk Factors For Developing Bladder Control Issues

STRUCTURAL CHALLENGES:

The female pelvic floor has less structural strength than the male pelvic floor, because the pelvic muscles are interrupted by three openings: the vagina, the urethra and the anus. This gender specific construction affects the conatinuity and strength of the female pelvic floor of muscles.

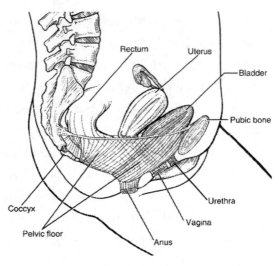

LIFE STAGE CHALLENGES:

Pregnancy and childbirth put added stress on pelvic muscles and on the bladder and its support structures. Women who have vaginal deliveries are at a higher risk of pelvic floor injury or weakness. The incident rates go even higher for women who have had multiple children or delivered large babies.

Menopause results in a decrease in estrogen, the female hormone. Estrogen contributes to pelvic muscle and urethral strength. A decrease in estrogen can affect the strength of the supporting tissues for the bladder and the urethra's ability to close completely.

OTHER CHALLENGES:

Surgeries and injuries of the bladder, urethra, brain, spinal cord, rectum or other pelvic organs may interfere with bladder control.

Won't It Just Go Away?

There are some bladder control problems that are temporary, meaning that they are related to some other event or transient situation and will improve. Other types of incontinence are chronic or long term. The differences in these two types of incontinence are important in order for treatment to be effective.

TEMPORARY BLADDER CONTROL ISSUES

The following are conditions or situations that can contribute to temporary or *transient incontinence:*

- bladder infection (urinary tract infection or "UTI")
- bladder stones
- some medications
- confusion or delirium
- restricted mobility
- depression
- dryness of the vagina and urethra (lack of estrogen)
- severe constipation
- large urine output (from diuretic medication)
- congestive heart failure
- diabetes or protein (kidney disease) in the urine
- pregnancy

If you are losing control of your bladder due to any of the aforementioned conditions, correcting the causative problem may relieve the symptoms. For example, treatment of a bladder infection can relieve incontinence. When permissible, changing a medication may make all the difference. Once a confused patient with pneumonia and a high fever is no longer delirious, the incontinence stops. Relieving severe constipation and reducing the pressure of the stool on the bladder and urethra can sometimes help urinary incontinence. Applying estrogen can improve the dryness and elasticity of the urethra.

Bottom line is it is so important to tell your health provider all of your symptoms, so he or she can start working with you to provide the appropriate treatment. For additional information, complete the assessment and severity index in Appendix 1 and give it to your health care provider as a tool to begin a dialogue about your pelvic health and fitness.

CHRONIC BLADDER CONTROL ISSUES

Loss of bladder control that is not related to a temporary situation is known as *chronic*. While there are numerous risk factors and causes of chronic incontinence, we will discuss the most common problems. Our hope is that the more you know, the greater your chances of minimizing or even eliminating your symptoms.

Types of Incontinence

Incontinence is classified as either **stress, urge, mixed or overflow.** Each category has specific causes and effective treatments.

STRESS INCONTINENCE

Stress urinary incontinence (SUI) is the most common form of incontinence. While its name implies otherwise, the cause of this type of incontinence is not stress related.

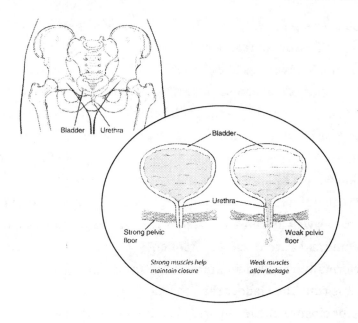

Stress incontinence occurs when the pressure in the bladder becomes too great for the bladder to withstand. It usually occurs because the pelvic floor muscles which support the bladder outlet are weakened. Urine tends to leak most when you cough, laugh or exercise jumping or running. In these situations, there is sudden pressure (stress) inside the abdomen and on the bladder. Varying amounts of urine may leak. The most common reason for the pelvic floor muscles to become weakened is childbirth. Stress incontinence is common in women who have had several children. It is also more common with increasing age and obesity. The good news about SUI is that non-invasive approaches such as pelvic floor exercise can usually be very helpful in lessening symptoms (see Chapter 3).

URGE INCONTINENCE

Urge incontinence (UI) is the involuntary loss of urine associated with a strong urge or desire to go to the bathroom. Though urge incontinence is the second most common form of bladder control problems, it remains a bit of a mystery. It is unclear why the bladder signals it is full when it is not (that "gotta go, gotta go" feeling). The woman feels a strong and sudden urge to go to the bathroom. Many times she cannot delay the urge and the unexpected result is embarrassing leakage. Environmental situations such as stepping out into the cold, being near the freezer section of the grocery store, hearing or seeing or touching water, arriving home and knowing a toilet is near, or conversely, being on a trip and knowing a toilet is not near might act as stimuli.

Frequent urination at night is also associated with urge incontinence, as well as going to the bathroom 20 to 30 times a day, but with minimal output (called "frequency").

Normally, the bladder stores urine until it receives a message that it is full. The bladder then contracts, the sphincters responsible for closure open, and urine is eliminated. If one is not in a socially acceptable place to urinate, this message can be ignored and going to the bathroom can be delayed for awhile. These messages are relayed from the bladder, through the spinal cord, to the brain and back to the bladder and sphincters. Anything that disrupts the nerve paths carrying these messages can interfere with the bladder function and cause symptoms of urgency or bladder over-activity. Simply, it means the person senses the need to go to the toilet but cannot get there in time to avoid leakage.

It is not uncommon for a person with urge symptoms to be in the bathroom every 45 to 60 minutes. It can be extremely disruptive to one's lifestyle.

> Nine out of ten cases of urinary incontinence are either stress or urge incontinence.

Mixed Incontinence
Symptoms include both stress and urge incontinence.

OVERFLOW INCONTINENCE

Finally, when the bladder becomes too full, it leaks small amounts of urine. Common in older people, the normal bladder-emptying mechanism becomes faulty. Without warning, one is unaware he/she needs to urinate.

What About Nighttime Trips to the Bathroom?

Nocturia in adults refers to being awakened at night with the need to go to the bathroom. *Noct* is a prefix pertaining to the night, *uria* pertains to urination. Nocturia is a common clinical complaint of adults. Nocturia is age-related and is frequently seen in otherwise healthy elderly women. For persons under the age of 65, it is considered normal to awaken zero to one time at night to urinate. For those over the age of 65, it is considered normal to get up one to two times a night. Getting up at night more than twice nightly is generally considered nocturia. It is not the same as nocturnal enuresis which refers to leaking urine during sleep.

It is important to diagnose true nocturia. True nocturia refers to being awakened because of the urge to go to the bathroom. It does not refer to the situation when a person is awakened by some other cause, be it pain, insomnia or a noise disturbance and then, incidentally she goes to the bathroom. Getting up to go the bathroom for whatever reason can eventually become a habit.

Not only is nocturia annoying, but it can result in sleep deprivation, fatigue, and traumatic injury from falls while navigating to the bathroom at night. Often the symptom presented to the physician is daytime tiredness or nighttime insomnia. Urinary frequency with discomfort may indicate inflammation of the bladder. Urinary frequency without discomfort may indicate excessive fluid intake, diabetes, congestive heart failure or a medication effect.

Factors leading to nocturia can be singular or multi-layered. With nocturia, there are three basic underlying factors: 1) the volume of urine output can increase during the night; 2) the bladder capacity can diminish during hours of sleep and 3) a combination. Forty-three percent of those with nocturia have an overproduction of urine at night. This is more common in the elderly. The circadian rhythm of the antidiuretic hormone may be altered affecting the amount of urine made at specific times of the 24-hour period. The filtration rate of the kidney may decrease affecting how much fluid is conserved. The cardiovascular system may not be able to pump enough blood to the kidneys during waking hours. When the latter occurs, more blood flows to the kidneys during sleep, causing more urine to be made while at rest. Specific causes of the nocturia are as follows: cardiovascular disease, diabetes, lower urinary tract obstruction or urinary retention, stroke, peripheral edema, unstable bladder, diuretic medications taken near bedtime, caffeine, alcohol or increased consumption of fluids at bedtime. An overactive bladder with a diminished capacity at nighttime can be caused by anxiety, bladder stones, cancer of the bladder or urethra, cystitis or medications.

EVALUATION

It is important to see your doctor or practitioner to establish the cause of nocturia. A medical history should be taken along with a physical examination. A 24-hour voiding diary is a helpful record of how much urine is being excreted at night providing an estimate of the bladder's capacity. This helps categorize the nocturia as increased urine output, overactive bladder or a combination of the two. Fluid intake patterns, medications, past surgery and other disease conditions should be considered. Signs of diabetes and congestive heart failure should be analyzed. Diagnostic tests to look at function disorders of the bladder are also performed, if necessary.

Treatment Options for Nocturia

Bladder problems are not always the cause of nocturia. Therefore, an accurate diagnosis is paramount when deciding a course of treatment. For example, if the cause is congestive heart failure and peripheral edema (fluid collecting in the legs), the treatment should address the congestive heart failure and the edema. Fluid management behaviors can be helpful. Restricting salt intake can help reduce fluid retention. Diuretics may be given in the middle to late afternoon so that they take effect before bedtime. Lying down for an hour or so before dinner helps to eliminate some of the accumulated fluid in the legs. Wearing compression hose or stockings throughout the day can also help minimize fluid build-up in the lower legs.

Dietary modification to avoid bladder irritants such as alcohol and caffeine can be helpful to those who suffer with nocturia. Training the bladder to hold more urine is appropriate for treating an overactive bladder. Strengthening the pelvic floor muscle is a part of the training process. Increase time between voids by fifteen-minute intervals to increase bladder capacity. At nighttime, try to resist the first urge and go back to sleep. With the next urge, get up and go to the bathroom. Try to suppress the next urge, and so on. For example, if you are getting up four or five times a night, try to decrease the interruption to two or three times, then two or one.

Medications may be effective in treating nocturia. Use of an antidiuretic hormone is an option with adults. The person must be monitored for symptoms such as headache or lightheadedness which might suggest electrolyte depletion. Side effects are rare in children but may occur in the elderly, especially those with congestive heart failure. Anticholinergic medications may be used in cases of bladder overactivity (See Chapter Seven). These can be effective in inhibiting bladder contractility and in increasing the bladder capacity.

Getting Help: Who to See

According to the National Association of Continence, many people with bladder control issues are too embarrassed to mention it to anybody, even their doctor. Educating the public about bladder and pelvic health is mandatory. Reassurance, effective treatment and impressive cure statistics will bring hope to those who feel hopeless.

Tell your doctor, nurse or physical therapist if you leak urine on a regular basis. They will assess your symptoms and present your treatment options. Sometimes a specialist, such as an urologist, urogynecologist or pelvic floor physical therapist is consulted.

In some situations, you and your doctor may decide to wait and see how things progress before embarking on any treatment. This is because some mild cases, such as post-partum incontinence, resolve themselves on their own.

UROGYNECOLOGISTS

Urogynecologists are either urologists or gynecologists who have specific training in the management of female pelvic disorders, including complex surgeries. Some urogynecologists specialize in the treatment of incontinence.

UROLOGISTS

Urologists are physicians who treat diseases of the urinary tract in women and the urinary and sex organs in men.

GYNECOLOGISTS

Gynecologists are doctors who specialize in the treatment of the female reproductive system. Some gynecologists perform diagnostic urological testing in their offices.

Nurses

Physicians will typically have nurses working with them who are familiar with the conservative treatment options. This includes the fitting of a pessary or catheter. Many nurses working in this field have specialized training and certification in the field of urology, wound or skin care and continence training. The nurses record personal histories and will often perform basic tests such as biofeedback.

Nurse Practitioners

A nurse practitioner is defined as a registered nurse who has received specialized training and certification. They are familiar with chronic incontinence and have the ability to order diagnostic tests and medications in most states. Most nurse practitioners can insert and care for pessaries and devices, can treat incontinence with electrical stimulation, can do biofeedback, will perform much of the diagnostic testing and, sometimes, will perform the initial physical exam. In many states, they are able to practice without the supervision of a physician.

Pelvic Floor Physical Therapists

Called "pelvic floor PT's," this group of care givers is first trained as general physical therapists and then go on for additional training in pelvic floor disorders for women and men. They provide treatments such as pelvic floor stimulation, biofeedback, massage and external/internal muscle and nerve work.

For information or to find any of the aforementioned health care providers, see References and Resources in the back of the book.

Now you know who to see if you have symptoms of bladder control problems. Let us now consider the various treatment options.

Facts about Bladder Control: Truth or Myth?

TRUTH OR MYTH

Please identify each statement below as Truth or Myth.

1. _____ Loss of bladder control is a normal part of aging.

2. _____ More women than men have symptoms of incontinence.

3. _____ Pregnancy and childbirth increase the risk of incontinence.

4. _____ Medications can contribute to loss of bladder control.

5. _____ After menopause, a woman cannot get help for incontinence.

Correct answers: 1. False, 2. True, 3. True, 4. True, 5. False

CHAPTER THREE

Exercises For A Better Bladder

Introducing the Pelvic Pyramid

Up until now, when someone used the words "incontinence" and "exercise" in the same breath, they were talking about "Kegels", exercises developed by a physician for the muscles of the pelvic floor. The pelvic floor is important for bladder control, for pelvic health and fitness. But it is only part of the solution. There are actually three sets of muscles essential in achieving and maintaining total pelvic health and stability, the muscles of the **Pelvic Pyramid**[4].

> The Pelvic Pyramid consists of the pelvic floor muscles (PFM), the transverse abdominals (TVA), and the multifidus. Think of it as "floor, plus core."

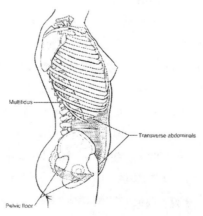

---

4   *The Pelvic Girdle*, Lee D. Churchill Livingstone: London, 1989.

The PFM are often described as a hammock that holds up the bladder, urethra and rectum organs. They serve as the base of your Pelvic Pyramid. The TVA muscle is like a corset around your abdomen that helps stabilize the pelvis and spine before movement. It is the front of your Pelvic Pyramid. The multifidus are a group of spider web-like muscles running from vertebra to vertebra, starting at your sacrum and running up to the mid-thoracic part of your spine (between your shoulder blades). It serves as the back of your Pelvic Pyramid. Working your Pelvic Pyramid regularly and correctly can improve bladder control and your sex drive, diminish back pain and even help you sleep through the night. So how do you do get started?

Introducing Total Control™

A new fitness and educational program was created by a team of nationally recognized urogynecologists, physical therapists and fitness experts to help women with bladder control and other pelvic floor dysfunctions. Called Total Control™, this innovative program enables women to locate, activate and work the muscles of the Pelvic Pyramid. Thereafter, a full body fitness program addresses common issues for all women, such as thoracic immobility, balance and weakness in other key stabilizing muscles.

The first lesson to learn in Total Control™ is how to isolate and contract the muscles of the Pelvic Pyramid without relying on other muscles to do the work or holding your breath.

You will learn to sustain the contraction for extended periods of time even during other stabilization exercises.

You also will learn how to contract the TVA, multifidus and pelvic floor muscles as a unit in different positions. We say "Engage Your Pelvic Pyramid" almost like a mantra. Engage your Pelvic Pyramid when you lift, sit, stand, walk or hold your baby. All are opportunities to exercise. Why? Because by being strong and stable in this core, you can eliminate symptoms of incontinence or prevent them from happening in the first place.

Clinical research has shown that Total Control™ can significantly improve or alleviate symptoms of both stress and urge incontinence. We are going to share some of the beginning exercises from Total Control™ below after a discussion of each individual muscle of the Pelvic Pyramid and include your daily beginning prescription.

For more information on the program and the fitness DVD, go to www.totalcontrolprogram.com. Remember, to think "**floor, plus core.**" First we will learn about the pelvic floor, then the transverse abdominals and finally, the multifidus.

The Floor of the Pelvic Pyramid: The Pelvic Floor

In preparing to do pelvic floor muscle work, the first thing women ask is, "What exactly am I supposed to be squeezing?" To that end, let us start with a definition and then take a look at the pelvic floor.

WHAT AND WHERE ARE THE PELVIC FLOOR MUSCLES?

Pelvic floor muscles are the muscles in the pelvis that join with connective tissue (fasciae and ligaments) to support the bladder, rectum, urethra and uterus. The muscles are woven around the urethra like a web. Because the urethra has to close tightly to keep urine from leaking, the muscles around the urethra need to be strong. These muscles also support your internal organs.

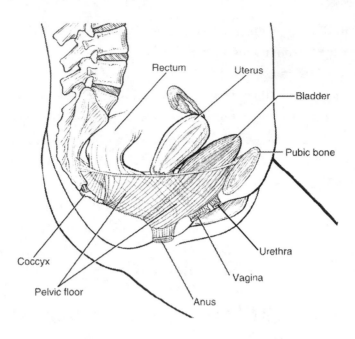

Rectum   Uterus

Bladder

Pubic bone

Coccyx

Urethra

Pelvic floor

Vagina

Anus

Think of the floor like the foundation for the home. The pelvic floor muscles span the area between the sides of the pelvic bone. Just as electrical and plumbing lines run through a house floor framing, blood vessels and nerves run through the tissues of the pelvic floor. When you are standing, this floor of muscle support is similar to a brand-new hammock in that it gives with weight, has the ability to stretch, but provides good support. An older and well-used hammock may tend to stretch and sag under weight. After pregnancy and childbirth, or with obesity, the pelvic floor muscles in women tend to relax and sag. Few women actually learn to correctly exercise and rehabilitate this group of muscles, even though there may have been significant stretching and/or injury during the pregnancy, labor and delivery. Maintaining muscle tone and strength in these supportive tissues is very important for bladder control.

There are two types of muscle fibers in the pelvic floor muscle group. Type I, or long muscle fibers, make up 70% of the muscle group and are responsible for sustained contractions. Type II, or short muscle fibers, make up the other 30% and are responsible for quick contractions such as those needed right before you sneeze. Think of the muscle fibers like runners, the long fibers being the distance runners (time and endurance) and the short fibers the sprint runners (fast and short acting). Both are needed for different circumstances of urinary control. Therefore, both should be strengthened.

WHY DO YOUR PELVIC FLOOR EXERCISES?

- Contracting (squeezing) the pelvic floor muscle helps to close the urethra so that the urine does not leak. This is important when there is pressure on the bladder, during coughing or lifting.
- Contracting these muscles also helps decrease the feeling of urgency. The pelvic floor muscles send a message to the bladder muscle (the detrusor) that the bladder should be in "holding" mode, as opposed to an "emptying" mode.
- Contracting the pelvic floor muscles builds strength for lifetime support of the pelvic organs. Women who have weak muscles are at higher risk for prolapse (a "fallen" bladder or uterus).
- Contracting these muscles improves your posture. The pelvic floor muscles are the floor of the Pelvic Pyramid. When energized, or engaged, with the other two muscles (TVA and multifidus), they can assist you in standing straight and tall.
- Contracting these muscles improves blood flow to the area. Improved blood flow can improve general tissue health and heighten sexual response.

HOW DO YOU STRENGTHEN YOUR PELVIC FLOOR MUSCLES?

Any muscle gets stronger through use, exercise and resistance. A muscle that is not used loses size, tone and strength. Move it or lose it! If you have ever had a cast on your leg or arm or were unable to use a limb because of injury or surgery, you probably noticed that the size of the muscle decreased from lack of use. The pelvic floor muscles keep some tone because they are constantly supporting the pelvic and abdominal organs. But they do not develop optimum strength and endurance without active exercise and intentional contractions. Endurance is related to strength. Strength is the capacity of the muscle to contract; endurance is how long the muscle can maintain a contraction. Both strength and endurance are needed to help with bladder support and control.

Since the muscles in your pelvis go around your urethra, vagina and rectum, an effective contraction of these muscles is a motion of lifting up and in your body. It is not a pushing-down movement. Many women have the tendency to also contract the muscles of the abdomen, thighs or buttocks when trying to contract the pelvic muscles. When doing your PFM exercises, focus on keeping those muscles relaxed.

To help you perform a PFM contraction, or "Kegel," concentrate on which muscles you should be using. Remember, these are internal muscles, there is not going to be anything visibly moving as you perform your squeezes or lifts. Going back to our hammock analogy, we want to lift the pelvic floor muscles up and in, thinking about that hammock becoming taut. Think about trying to stop a stream of urine or from passing gas. Because we want to draw up and in, some women think about gently drawing a tampon into their vaginas. We like to imagine a tampon made out of crystal to prevent any massive grabbing sensation. With every analogy, you do want to think "gentle" to prevent yourself from using other muscles, such as the abdomen during your workout.

Position is pivotal to pelvic floor training. It helps insure successful involvement of the proper muscles.

The Front of the Pelvic Pyramid: Transverse Abdominals (TVA)

Now let us move to the front of our Pelvic Pyramid and look at the transverse abdominals (transversus abdominus in Latin) or the "TVA." As with the pelvic floor, it can be helpful to take a look at the areas in question.

WHAT AND WHERE IS MY TVA?

Your transverse abdominal is underneath those six-pack abs you are cultivating at the gym. You just might not have ever *tried* to work them. The TVA is the deepest abdominal muscle. It helps to hold your spine and pelvis stable. It works with the other Pelvic Pyramid muscles to support the organs of the pelvis. Strong TVA muscles can also give you a flat tummy.

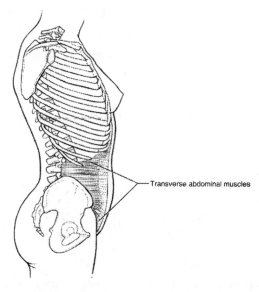

Transverse abdominal muscles

Most people spend quite a bit of time in their fitness regime focusing on their "abs," their rectus abdominals and obliques. Both of these muscle groups play their roles in having us look great in our bathing suit. But it is the *transverse abdominal* that rule the world of continence. Your TVA runs from front to back and is a primary support for both the spine and the pelvis. To effectively work your TVA, you first need to be in a proper body position.

How To Work The TVA

GET IN AN OPTIMAL POSITION: NEUTRAL SPINE

While there are many positions for good TVA work, we recommend that you start on your back in a "hooklying position", which is with knees bent, feet flat on the floor. Keep your buttocks and thighs relaxed and find your neutral spine by first flattening your low back to the floor. This will put you in a slight pelvic tilt. Next, rock your pelvis the opposite direction, sending your tailbone to the floor which will, in turn, make your low back arch *off* the floor. Do this a few times in each direction, rocking and rolling through your pelvic range of motion, front to back. Now settle into a comfortable place somewhere in between. This is the place where your buttocks are on the floor and resting. You should feel equal weight distribution of both sides of your pelvis and between your shoulder blades. You might be able to reach underneath your low back and feel a little space at about your waistline. This is **your neutral spine.** To work TVA, you need to keep your back in a neutral position and remain relaxed.

RIB CAGE (DIAPHRAMATIC) BREATHING:

It is important to work your TVA muscles with diaphragmatic or rib cage breathing while in neutral spine. To do this, place your hands on either side of your ribcage. Take a slow, medium size inhale and try to breathe out through your hands and through the back of your body. Continue taking some breaths, focusing on expanding out and into your hands, as opposed to your tummy. This is harder than it sounds. If the exercise is done properly, your belly will remain quiet and only your ribcage will be moving. Practice this a few more times.

Find Your TVA Landmarks:

There is a spot on your low stomach where you have a good chance of actually feeling this gentle abdominal work. In Total Control™, we encourage "touch learning" to keep your brain in the game. With TVA work, in particular, keeping your fingers on your landmarks can be very helpful to get the right muscles to work *and* to know if you are recruiting some of your other, more dominant ab muscles. So, here we go...

Using your index and middle fingers, locate the top of your hip bones. Find the TVA muscle by moving the flat fingertips two to three inches toward the center of your body and two to three inches down toward the pubic bone. We are at the top of a low-rise bikini. This is the place you want to keep your fingers, flat on the skin—remember we are not excavating; we're just keeping our brains in the game by having our fingers here.

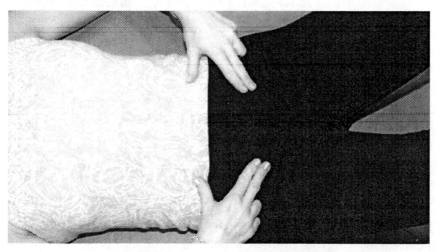

This is a place where you have the "possibility" of feeling a TVA contraction. Do not get discouraged if at first you don't feel anything. Remember, these are deep, deep muscles. Many women work for weeks on TVA before they feel the muscles working. Trust us, you *do* have them and they will work with proper positioning and concentration.

Think "Gentle":

The feeling of a good TVA contraction is subtle, a slight tensing of the muscle fibers under your fingertips. Your pelvis should be still and your buttocks and thighs relaxed. This is not a forceful or big movement. Instead, the sensation is as if the muscles were pulling away from your fingers. *You should not feel a bulge.*

Use visualizations to activate TVA:

Here are three visualizations we use in Total Control™:

- Imagine zipping up tight, low-rise jeans that have a delicate, silk zipper. We say zip versus button, because we do not want you to pelvic tilt under to get that top button buttoned.
- Imagine a birthday candle held over your low belly. Gently draw your navel away from it.
- Imagine a corset running from back to front around your low waist. Think about gently tightening the corset underneath your fingers.

> We always want to stress the word "gentle" with TVA work. This is not "the burn" of abs of steel. If you try to force a hard contraction, your big bully muscle, rectus (on top) and obliques (on the sides), get involved. Think gentle, gentle, gentle.

The Back of the Pelvic Pyramid: The Multifidus

Finally, we will complete our Pelvic Pyramid by getting to know our multifidus muscle (technically, a group of spider web-like muscles or "multifidi," but we will use the singular version). The multifidus works with its other two counterparts; front and floor. It is hidden from our view by some large skeletal muscles on top.

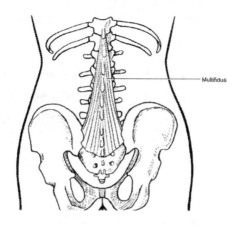

Multifidus

WHAT AND WHERE IS MY MULTIFIDUS?

Your multifidus muscle is underneath your big back muscles, erector spinae, running from vertebra to vertebra, starting at your sacrum and running up to the mid-thoracic spine (between your shoulder blades). This muscle is your back's best friend, because when it is strong, it allows the lower back to work without pain. The multifidus muscle facilitates all bending and twisting, so you want to take care of the back of your Pelvic Pyramid.

How To Work The Multifidus

1. GET IN AN OPTIMAL POSITION: SIDE-LYING

To best feel multifidus working, you again will want to take gravity out of the picture and use "touch learning" to bring your brain into the game and feel this subtle muscle work.

> We recommend doing multifidus isolation with a prop of a 6" ball (from the Total Control™ class kit) or a small hand towel folded over in thirds under your foot or ankle.

Lie on one side with your hips stacked. Bend your bottom leg at the knee, with the top leg positioned so as to bisect the area from the knee to the foot of the bottom leg. The top ankle will rest on your ball or folded towel. Your legs will be forming a figure "four."

Your hips must remain aligned and your spine should be in a comfortable neutral spine position.

2. Always Engage Tva When Working Multifidus

Whenever you are on your side, you will want to be conscious of engaging your TVA muscles prior to activating other muscles groups. The multifidus is no exception. You stand a better chance activating and feeling multifidus work with your transverse energized.

3. Find Your Spinal Valleys

There is an optimal spot to touch to potentially feel multifidus engagement. Reach back and, with your top hand, place three to four fingers on one side of your spine at about your waistline. In this muscular valley, on either side of your bony spine, you might be able to feel a gentle "puffing" or swelling of the multifidus muscles when you start the exercises.

4. Use Visualizations To Activate Multifidus

Here are three visualizations we use in Total Control™:

- Imagine your spine getting long from the tailbone downward.
- Imagine trying to separate the vertebrae of your low back, as if they were a candy necklace with elastic in between.
- Imagine arching your tailbone back to touch the back of your head. *(Note: This is obviously impossible. It is simply something to visualize)*

5. Think Gentle Pressure:

To begin multifidus work, press down slightly into the pillow or onto the ball, there will be no large movements of your spine. You may feel a swelling or bulging underneath your fingers. If you feel a muscular twitch, that is a good start. Continue to work at feeling the slight swelling and bulging under your finger tips.

Now that you have these introductions into positions and sensations, breathing and visualizations, let's specifically begin to "Energize Your Pelvic Pyramid!" For our session, you will need a small hand towel or a 6" Total Control™ ball, comfortable clothing and a mat or towel for the floor.

Daily Exercises For Your Pelvic Pyramid: Floor, Plus Core

1. SIDE-LYING PELVIC FLOOR EXERCISE:

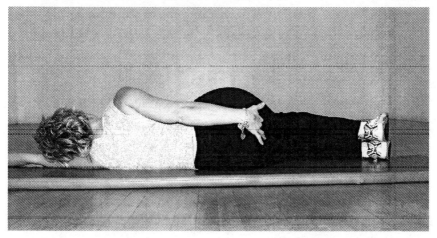

Purpose: To work pelvic floor muscles in an optimal position, without gravity, and to potentially feel the sensation of the muscles working

HOW TO'S:

- Lying down with your legs bent and drawn up comfortably (about a 45- degree angle from your hip joint to your knee), rest your head on your bottom arm
- Take the second and third fingers of the hand of your top arm and reach them back along your spine and down to the bony end of your tailbone

- Now, reach between your legs, keeping your knees bent and relaxed, until you get to your perineum—the space between your anus and vagina. Keep your fingers here during the exercise and see if you can feel any movement beneath your fingers
- Breathe normally and keep breathing throughout the exercise
- Remember your analogies: holding back urine, hammock, tampon

Daily Prescription:

- In a "waltz" tempo, perform a one count contraction followed by a two count relaxation for a series of 10 short holds. Think "lift, off, off," or "on, off, off." Rest for 10 second in between sets
- Immediately follow this "waltz" series with 10 sets of a sustained hold of 10 - 15 seconds. After each hold, rest for the same amount of time you hold (i.e. 10 second rest after a 10 second hold)

Common Mistakes:

- Tilting the pelvis, holding your breath, using your bottom, abs or inner thighs

To develop strength in your pelvic muscles, you need to plan an exercise program. Just like any exercise program, goals need to be set, a protocol followed, effort consistently maintained.

You can break up your training and do five waltz sets and five sustained holds in the morning and five and five in the evening before you go to bed.

2. Hook-lying Pelvic Floor Exercise:

Beginner's Position

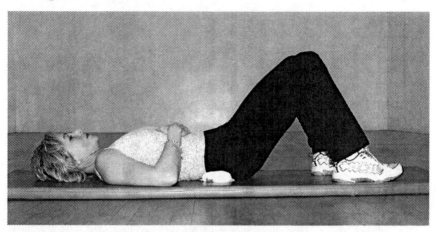

Advanced Position

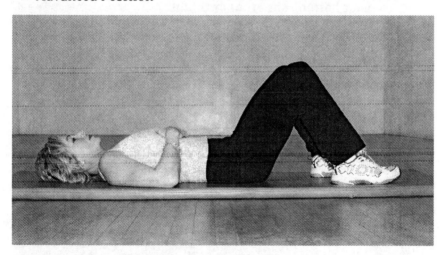

Purpose: To work pelvic floor muscles in another optimal position, minimizing gravity to facilitate feeling the sensation of the muscles working

How To's:

- ◦ Lying down on your back, have your knees comfortably bent and feet placed on the floor
- ◦ Keep all other muscles quiet as you think "up & in"

- Remember to keep breathing and breathe normally throughout the exercise
- Remember your analogies: holding back urine, hammock, tampon

DAILY PRESCRIPTION:

- In a "waltz" tempo, perform 10 short holds. Think "lift, off, off," or "on, off, off." Rest for 10 second in between sets
- Lift and hold for a sustained hold of 10 - 15 seconds x 10 sets. After each hold, rest for the same amount of time you hold (i.e. 10 second rest after a 10 second hold)

COMMON MISTAKES:

- Tilting the pelvis; holding your breath; using other muscles, like your bottom, abs or inner thighs

  When you first do this exercise, roll up a small hand towel and place it underneath your tailbone. This puts you in a slight pelvic tilt and takes weight off your pelvic floor. It is easier to feel the muscles working. Once you have mastered "feeling it" with the towel, take it away & lie flat on the floor.

3. TRANSVERSE ABDOMINAL (TVA):

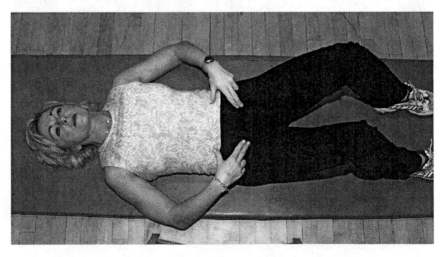

Purpose: To locate and perform an isolated contraction of the transverse abdominals with the activation of other stomach muscles

How To's:

- Lie down on the floor with your knees comfortably bent and feet flat on the floor
- Find your TVA landmarks, 2 - 3 inches down and in from your hipbones & keep your fingers lightly pressing onto your abdomen
- Using your ribcage breathing and maintaining neutral spine, use your favorite visualization and perform short and sustained holds. Inhale ribcage, exhale & engage TVA
- Remember it is a gentle contraction

Daily Prescription:

- Perform 6 - 8 short holds
- Finish with sustained holds, 8 - 10 reps for 10 - 20 seconds. Remember to rib cage BREATHE throughout the sustained hold

Common Mistakes:

- Creasing at the waist (means other abdominals are taking over), excessive rib movement, flattening the navel to the ground, tensing your bottom or pressing out your abdomen

  Be patient! Sometimes it takes the TVA muscles 10 to 20 seconds to respond. The goal is to feel the engagement right away and to hold it for 10 seconds or more. If your TVA muscles are twitching, keep your fingers still. Some people can do this exercise right away, but most of us need days or even weeks before it starts to come easily.

4. MULTIFIDUS:

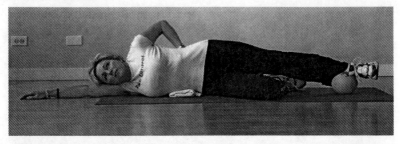

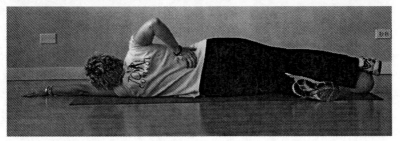

Purpose: To locate and perform an isolated contraction of the multifidus with the activation of other back muscles

HOW TO'S:

- Lie on your side, hips stacked.
- Engage TVA
- Bend your bottom leg, with the top leg positioned so as to bisect the area from the knee to the foot of the bottom leg. Making a figure "four" with your legs. The top ankle will rest on a 6" ball or folded towel.
- Your spine should be in a comfortable neutral spine position
- Find your multifidus landmark, the valley to the side of your spine
- Gently press down on the ball
- Think of your analogies, getting long from your tailbone down or trying to imagine touching your tailbone to the back of your head

Daily Prescription:

- Perform 6 - 8 short holds
- Finish with one sustained hold 10 seconds
- Switch sides and repeat

Common mistakes:

- Rolling backward or forward in the hips or not engaging the TVA muscles

A Testimonial to Total Control™

Thank you for the privilege of being part of your Total Control™ Program. This program gave me far more than I had hoped for and some of the benefits were a total surprise!

When I entered your group, I was seeing a therapist for serious depression due to my problems with incontinence. The condition so horrified me that I did not even tell my therapist or anyone else until I entered your class. I did tell a doctor who gave me a prescription which I never filled. I did not want to mask my symptoms with chemicals. I *did not know* that holistic help was available.

So I had become a recluse. I was depressed, and I became inactive. I did not know what to do, so I did nothing. I had given up. I was waiting to die. I am 72 years old. I thought that my time was coming to an end. Then, by coincidence, I found out about your group and thought it sounded special.

Through this group, I learned the cause of my incontinence and what I could do to help myself. I gained control. My depression lifted and, surprisingly, I felt very alive. I am filled with hope and a strong desire to be productive again. I still do have a lot to offer.

My therapy ended, and my therapist was impressed with my progress. My daughter was so impressed with the changes in me that she offered to pay for any advanced classes.

You saved my life. I am so grateful. I cannot thank you enough.

Carol, 72; Chicago

CHAPTER FOUR

How You Live Matters

Bladder Friendly (Or Not) Lifestyle Traits

In addition to exercise, how we live our lives can improve our pelvic health. In this chapter, we will look at lifestyle issues, areas of personal behavior that can have an impact on bladder control. We will discuss nutrition and constipation to show their impact on pelvic health. In Chapter Five, we will look at biofeedback and simple devices that can give us a holistic perspective.

There are a few lifestyle habits that might increase the risk of incontinence. As we strive to be dry, it is important to recognize them. They include the following:

SMOKING

Smoking can actually affect urinary incontinence in three ways:

1. Nicotine can be a bladder "irritant" which causes the bladder to be more active, a situation that contributes to urge incontinence.

2. A smoker may have a chronic cough that increases abdominal pressure, weakening the bladder and urethral supports and contributing to stress incontinence.

3. Smoking can decrease the blood supply to the bladder by causing narrowing of the arteries.

WEIGHT

Obesity (excessive body mass) can increase the risk of both stress incontinence and urge incontinence. The extra weight of obesity increases the stress on the pelvic floor muscles. These muscles support the pelvic organs (bladder, urethra and uterus) and the abdominals when we are upright. Weight loss can reduce the pelvic pressure and lessen some of the stress. It can improve the symptoms of stress incontinence for some. Overweight women also have an increased risk for urge incontinence. Not fully understood, the problem might be the result of the increased abdominal pressure. New studies indicate a direct correlation between weight loss and improvement in bladder control. A current NIH funded, multi-site study is studying this further.

So, weight loss is a definite contributing factor of stress incontinence in women. Exercise specifically devoted to pelvic floor muscles is very important to bladder control. Total body fitness and good health should be goals.

EXERCISE

High-impact exercises (aerobics, jumping, jogging, physically active work or lifting) create more stress on the pelvic muscles and the support ligaments for the bladder. Additionally, crunches and other traditional abdominal exercises may exacerbate bladder control problems. The abdominal muscles contract with exertion, increasing pressure on the bladder. The pelvic floor muscles need to be able to counter this force. Research by Kari Bo from the Norwegian University of Sport and Physics concurs that high performance athletes, even young college-age women, need higher toned pelvic floors.[5] This finding confirms the importance of working the Pelvic Pyramid muscles.

---

5 "Female Elite Athletes Require Stronger Pelvic Floor Muscles to Prevent UI," K. Bo, *Women's Health Weekly*, 2004

Diet/fluid habits

Certain fluids and foods can be irritants to the lining of the bladder, causing the bladder to be sensitive and overactive. Some known bladder irritants are: alcohol, caffeine, coffee, tea, soda, chocolate, spicy foods, citrus fruits and juices, tomatoes and tomato products, sugars, medicines with caffeine and artificial sweeteners (aspartame).

The Impact of Other Conditions

There are several disease conditions that can affect bladder control for both males and females:

- **A stroke** can interrupt the nerve messages from the brain to the bladder that are responsible for bladder control.
- **Diabetes** can cause an increase in the amount of urine produced, resulting in sugar spilling over into the urine. It also can affect the nerves and blood vessels involved in bladder function.
- **Parkinson's disease** can affect messages from the brain needed for bladder control.
- **Alzheimer's disease or other types of dementia** can affect a person's ability to locate the toilet, even the purpose of a toilet.
- **Multiple sclerosis** affects the spinal cord and can interrupt the nerve messages as they travel through the spinal cord.
- **Certain types of cancer and/or radiation treatments** that involve organs in the pelvis, the brain, or spinal cord can affect bladder control. For example, treatment involving radiation to the pelvis for cancer of the cervix can affect the bladder and urethra, because they are located so close to the cervix. Inflammation and later scarring to the tissues can occur with radiation treatments. Cancer of the lung can

result in chronic coughing and, consequently, symptoms of stress incontinence.

- **Injuries** can be very similar to diseases in their impact. Injuries to the spinal cord, brain, bladder or pelvis may result in disruption of bladder control, depending on the areas affected. The actual organ may be injured or the nerves and blood vessels associated with that organ may be damaged, affecting the function of the organ.

The Effects of Aging

Contrary to popular myth, bladder control problems are not a normal part of aging. Not everyone will become incontinent. However, there are certain age-related changes or occurrences that can increase the risk of incontinence.

1. **Decreased muscle tone** - The bladder and pelvic floor muscles lose strength and tone. This would affect the ability of the bladder to contract and empty itself and the ability of the pelvic muscles to help the bladder sphincter close.

2. **Increased bladder contractions, but with less strength** - The bladder contracts more but with less effectiveness. It becomes more sensitive and hyperactive.

3. **Decreased sensation** - The nerves to the bladder are not as efficient as they once were at carrying a message. A person is not always aware of the need to go to the bathroom. The message is delayed, so there is less time to move safely to the toilet without leaking urine.

4. **Less mobility** - A person requires more time getting to the bathroom and/or removing clothing before urinating.

5. **Decreased heart contraction strength** - The heart is not as powerful a pump as it once was. Because it cannot keep the blood moving through the body with the same force, fluids

build up in the ankles and feet. This retention means there is less fluid available to circulate through the body and kidneys. Less urine is made. This can lead to increased urinary output at night.

6. **Taking many medications at one time** - Some drugs do not interact with each other and have side effects that affect bladder contractions. Examples are sedatives, pain medicines or antihistamines, allergy and cold remedies. The elderly are more likely to take multiple medications and should be very cautious.

7. **Co-existing ailments** - A person may suffer from more than one disease, resulting in many symptoms and medications. A physician or health care provider should be consulted.

A combination of therapies might be appropriate for a person with a myriad of bladder issues. Your physician needs to evaluate your case to determine the most appropriate treatment options. Keeping a 24-hour bladder diary is helpful.

Nutrition & Your Pelvic Health

Fluids

Why is fluid management important? Fluids are crucial to all functions of the body. The bladder is responsible for eliminating a great deal of those fluids.

Many persons with limited bladder control think that if they limit their fluid intake, they will go to the bathroom fewer times and have less urine leakage. It is true that the less we drink, the less the urine output. But this pattern may actually increase bladder control problems. If a person drinks too little, the body conserves fluids by decreasing what the kidney and bladder will eliminate. As a result, the amount of urine decreases and becomes stronger or more concentrated.

> Think of making a pitcher of lemonade from a powder packet. If you only add half of the recommended water to the pitcher, the lemonade will be stronger and more concentrated than if you added the recommended amount. By adding more water, you can dilute the lemonade.

Just as concentrated lemonade may make your mouth "pucker," strong or concentrated urine can make your bladder "pucker" or contract. The bladder can react with strong contractions even though it is not full of urine. The concentrated urine enters the bladder, serves as a "stimulant." The bladder contracts more actively than normal. Therefore, if you try to cut back on drinking fluids in an attempt to prevent leaking urine, you may actually experience more urgency and leakage. Fluids are needed to keep the urine from becoming too concentrated. Women with symptoms of urge incontinence (frequency, having to get to the bathroom in a hurry) or mixed incontinence need to drink water throughout the day rather than in large amounts at one time.

Fluid restriction may be appropriate at the end of the day, a few hours before bedtime. But all-day fluid restriction, unless advised by your health professional for some other condition, is not a healthy idea.

The preferred way to drink fluids, water being the best choice, is to drink small amounts of liquid throughout the day. Carrying a water bottle everywhere and sipping small amount continuously is actually a very good behavioral option for bladder control problems.

Note some medications contain caffeine and may be irritating to your bladder. These include, but are not limited to:

- Anacin
- Excedrin
- Vanquish
- Midol
- Coryban-D

- Dristan
- No-Doz & Vivarin

Not everyone is affected the same by these irritants. What bothers one woman may not affect another. You must be aware of your own reaction to various foods and drinks. One person reported an increase in urgency and frequency after ingesting Altoids, a common breath mint. If you suspect something bothers your bladder, eliminate that item for a few days to see if it makes a difference. If your bladder is sensitive, it may take a few days to make a difference. Even if you identify coffee, chocolate, lemonade or something else as an irritant, you do not necessarily have to permanently change your diet. But you may want to pay attention to the "timing" of your ingestion. For example, you consider your diet while on a plane ride or car trip, in the late afternoon, before a social function, before a long business meeting.

Some fluids act as diuretics, meaning they increase urine output. Known diuretics are water, beer, coffee, soda, watermelon, grapefruit juice and tea. Again, pay attention to your personal reactions to what you are drinking, and make your choices from that information. Again, be careful not to reduce your intake to a level that causes your body to conserve fluid and produce urine that is too concentrated. Six to eight glasses of water per day are generally recommended. If you are exercising, live in a dry and hot climate, or have a fever or diarrhea, increase your water intake.

> In a study of 450 female soldiers conducted by physicians in the Department of Obstetrics and Gynecology at Madigan Army Medical Center, Tacoma, WA, one third of the women experienced urinary incontinence during their exercise and field training activities. A disturbing fact was that thirteen percent of these women limited their fluid intake significantly to reduce their urinary symptoms.[6]

---

6   *Behavioral Treatment of Exercise-Induced Urinary Incontinence Among Female Soldiers,* Sherman RA, Davis Gd, Wang MF, 1997.

Limiting fluids, or self-dehydrating, during exercise can be very dangerous. Dehydration reduces urine output and can cause dizziness, confusion, irritability, heat exhaustion and even a coma. Extreme dehydration can lead to death. If you are exercising, maintain a healthy fluid intake. One rule of thumb is to drink enough fluids so that your urine is very lightly colored or almost clear.

CONSTIPATION

Constipation is quite common. You might wonder how this is relevant to urinary incontinence. Constipation, or hard formed stool in the rectum, can affect urinary function. If the rectum is filled, pressure and forward displacement of the bladder can occur. This can affect the ability of the bladder sphincter to close tightly and prevent urine from leaking. A large amount of stool in the rectum can prevent the bladder from emptying completely. Constipation can also aggravate an overactive bladder. Chronic straining (or bearing down) for a bowel movement can weaken the pelvic floor muscles, similar to pushing down on a hammock and stretching it. So, when the rectum fills with stool and a message is sent from the brain for evacuation, you should immediately act upon the urge. If it is chronically suppressed, the urge becomes less noticeable and more easily ignored.

Several things can contribute to constipation, either temporarily or chronically. Medications, lack of exercise, a diet low in fiber and fluids, travel, a change in routine and illness can all be factors. If you have chronic problems with bowel elimination, you should consult your health care provider. Begin a behavioral program for management of your bowels before you start a behavioral program for your bladder. This is important because your constipation can interfere with the effectiveness of your bladder program.

Helpful Hints for Constipation

1. Drink plenty of fluids
2. Eat grains, fruits and vegetables for fiber
3. Bran or fiber can be added to muffins, jams, cereal
4. Exercise daily
5. Try to establish a routine for bowel elimination
6. Respond to the urge for a bowel movement
7. Allow yourself plenty of time for evacuation
8. Avoid the use of laxatives, if possible
9. See a health care provider experienced in bowel training programs

Fiber

Dietary fiber is a group of substances found only in foods derived from plants. There are two major categories of fiber, soluble and insoluble which are thought to have different effects on health.

- **Soluble fiber**, found in fruits, oats, barley and some beans, dissolves in water and is degraded by bacteria in your colon. It increases stool volume and stool water content. Soluble fiber forms a gel in your intestines which regulates the flow of waste material throughout your digestive tract. It slows stomach-emptying time, delaying the absorption of glucose from your bloodstream and has been shown to lower cholesterol. Increasing dietary fiber intake, independent of fat intake, is an important dietary component for the prevention of fatal heart disease.

- **Insoluble fiber** passes through your digestive system largely unchanged. Examples are found in cereals, wheat bran and the stalks and peels of fruits and vegetables. The ingestion of vegetables helps protect us from both colorectal and breast cancer. Insoluble fiber accelerates intestinal transit, increases fecal weight, slows starch hydrolysis and delays glucose absorption. With larger, softer and more frequently moving feces, your intestinal walls are scoured and waste matter is removed. Experts believe this action reduces the risk for colorectal cancer and certain types of benign tumors.

Most Americans eat only about 10 grams of dietary fiber each day, when the suggested range for adults is 25-35 grams per day. Eating fiber-rich foods at each meal is ideal and easy, since fiber is found in a variety of food sources. If you are taking a supplement of individual fibers, we recommend that you tell your physician. Most importantly, when fiber intake is increased, water intake must be increased as well. You will know that you are consuming enough fiber and fluid when your stools are large and soft. We do not recommend reliance on laxative pills. Mineral oil is not advised either, because it substantially reduces the absorption of nutrients.

REGULARITY RECIPE

The following is a recipe for a high-fiber jam that can be made at home and kept in the refrigerator. Eating it with toast or crackers daily can help provide fiber to your diet and reduce constipation. It also may be helpful for symptoms of Irritable Bowel Syndrome.

HIGH FIBER JAM

1 cup applesauce
1 cup bran
½ cup prune juice

This mixture should have a jam-like consistency. Keep mixture refrigerated in a covered container.

Eat one tablespoon of the mixture every evening for a morning bowel movement. If you do not notice an improvement within a couple of days, increase your portion to two tablespoons every evening. For most people this is enough. However, if you are not experiencing regular bowel movements, you may add up to two tablespoons in the morning as well, up to a maximum of four. Always drink one large glass of water with the jam.

In Summary

By understanding bladder control, its causes and risk factors, you might be able to prevent or reduce incidents of incontinence. For example, if you leak urine when you laugh or cough, losing weight or practicing pelvic floor exercises might help relieve symptoms. If you experience urinary frequency, eliminate bladder irritants from your diet and change your bladder habits.

CHAPTER FIVE

Behavioral Treatments—Basic Training For The Bladder

This chapter discusses what every woman should know about pelvic health. Many of the tips and topics are common knowledge, or so we thought, until we began speaking with women everywhere about their bodies, their habits and their lives. We have compiled information about many of the treatment options, some simple and others more drastic. The data are interesting and the spectrum of treatment is vast. Having good bathroom habits or watching what we eat or drink can help us to stay in control.

TREATMENT OPTIONS

	Stress Incontinence	Urge Incontinence
Exercise	X	X
Diet	X	X
Bladder Training	X	X
Vaginal Cones	X	NO
Biofeedback	X	X
Electrical Stimulation	X	X
Pessaries (Pelvic Support Devices)	X	NO

Bladder Training

Bladder training sounds so simple you might minimize its importance in improving your symptoms. Remember, the bladder is a muscle and it works in response to a message sent by a nerve. To start any type of muscle/nerve training, you have to deliberately think, then act and practice. Eventually, the "think" part becomes almost subconscious and is more like a reaction. Remember when you learned to use a typewriter or a computer keyboard? Initially, every letter required concentration. After time and practice, the process became second nature. In like manner, the bladder can be trained to suppress an urge to empty, to hold more urine or to empty more completely.

Decide what symptoms are most bothersome. Do you want to go to the bathroom less frequently? Are you emptying your bladder every 45 minutes? Are you not sleeping well because of repeated trips to the bathroom during the night? Do you have to go to the bathroom every 15 minutes because you do not completely empty your bladder? Write down which bathroom habit you would like to change and then set goals for yourself. Record your progress weekly as you work on each point.

SYMPTOMS I HAVE

Example 1: *I have to go to the bathroom every waking hour.*

Example 2: *As soon as I walk into my house, I have to rush to the bathroom.*

1. _____

2. _____

3. _____

4. _____

5. _____

GOALS

Example 1: *I want to delay every bathroom visit by 15 minutes.*

Example 2: *I want to enter my home and wait 10 minutes before going to the toilet.*

1. _____

2. _____

3. _____

4. _____

5. _____

MY PROGRESS	
Week 1	**Week 2**
1. _____	1. _____
2. _____	2. _____
3. _____	3. _____
4. _____	4. _____
5. _____	5. _____
6. _____	6. _____
Week 3	**Week 4**
1. _____	1. _____
2. _____	2. _____
3. _____	3. _____
4. _____	4. _____
5. _____	5. _____
6. _____	6. _____

SALLY'S STORY

Sally is a 33-year-old mother of two. During the day, she has to urinate every 45 minutes, sometimes as often as every 15 minutes. At other times, she feels the need to urinate immediately after she empties her bladder. Sally is a professional in the health care field and finds this frequency to be very disruptive at work. She does not leak urine, but she starts to feel very uncomfortable if she does urinate often. She drinks several cups of coffee every morning and two to three sodas (diet/caffeine free) throughout the day. Sally sought help for her urinary frequency and was recommended for behavioral therapy.

Sally's first behavioral modification was her fluid intake. She gradually began to drink less coffee and soda and increase her water intake. Her goal was to reduce the fluid irritants to her bladder, making it less hyperactive.

Her next assignment was to practice letting her urge pass by waiting 15 minutes longer than usual before going to the bathroom. She was careful not to wait too long. Her goal was to gradually increase her bladder's capacity.

Sally started to see improvements within four weeks and was able to wait 2 hours between voids by 8 weeks. Her goal was to reach 2.5 hours. This may not seem significant, but for someone who was constantly thinking about the bathroom, this was a major accomplishment.

Urge Inhibition or Suppression

This process of gently "holding back" requires practice and time to succeed. Do not make the mistake of thinking that if you do this correctly one time, you will be safe. Until you are certain you have control, stay in a comfortable environment with a toilet nearby.

When you get an urge to urinate, take a deep breath. Relax. Then perform a quick pelvic muscle contraction, and let the urge pass. Distract yourself mentally if you can. Try a brief physical distraction such as making out a to-do list, straightening up your desk, or making a quick phone call. While you work, keep relaxing and take slow, deep breaths. This becomes easier with experience.

Wait a few minutes, and then slowly go to the toilet, squeezing your pelvic muscles as you walk. Rushing only makes the bladder more likely to contract more and increases your chance of an "accident," either leaking urine or falling.

Gradually increase the time between urinating. Start by waiting just five minutes, a two and one-half to three hour interval being optimum. It may take up to a week to see any progress. If you have severe urge symptoms, it may take even longer. Try not to get discouraged. Be patient and practice.

The Knack: "Squeeze Before You Sneeze"

The "Knack,"[7] called "squeeze before you sneeze," is a method used to retain bladder control when you cough or sneeze by first activating the pelvic floor muscles. Mastering the "Knack" will help support the urethra during times when there is pressure on the bladder.

WHEN SHOULD I USE MY PELVIC FLOOR MUSCLES?

You should contract your pelvic floor muscles whenever you anticipate pressure on your bladder, when lifting, coughing, or sneezing. You should also contract these muscles to delay going to the toilet and just after you have finished going to the toilet. You should *avoid* routinely stopping your urine midstream to contract your muscles.

It is important that you learn to breathe at the same time you contract the muscles so you can hold them steady during a cough or sneeze. **Practice holding the muscles contracted while breathing.** Steadily contracting the pelvic floor muscles while breathing in and out will seem unnatural at first, but you will be able to adjust.

Experiment with contracting the pelvic floor muscles in many different positions—standing upright, on hands and knees, feet together and apart, lying and sitting. Make the "Knack" a mindful habit and feel yourself gaining control.

---

7   "On Pelvic Floor Muscle Function and Stress Urinary Incontinence: Effects of Posture, Parity and Volitional Control," *In Nursing*, 1996: Ann Arbor: University of Michigan;, pgs 152-154.

A Word About "Just In Case" Peeing

As preschoolers, we were taught to go to the bathroom "just in case." This preventative peeing is detrimental to the health of your bladder muscles and can contribute to the feeling that you always have to go. Normal bladder function involves coordination between the brain and bladder. Contrary to what most of us think, properly voiding is a voluntary action. Ultimately, it is the brain, not the bladder that should be in charge. It is mind over bladder.

PROPER POSITION

To optimally void, there are two important elements:

1. Remember to sit down all the way with your legs apart. Do not hover. This will allow the bladder and urethra to properly expel urine.

2. Rushing through urination promotes "bearing down," which, as we have already noted, is hazardous to the long-term health of your pelvic floor muscles.

Rock 'N' Roll

If you feel that you are not emptying your bladder completely, try a technique we call, "Rock 'n' Roll." After you urinate, rock back and forth, or front to back, on the toilet seat. Because the bladder walls have crevices where urine can deposit, you may, in fact, have some residual urine after the first void. Do not push or strain.

Double Voiding

Double voiding is another technique to make sure you have completely emptied your bladder. After going to the bathroom once, relax and try to empty your bladder again, without "bearing down." Sometimes, you might want to stand up or just change positions in between the first and second urination.

Interestingly enough, many pregnant women double void intuitively, changing positions on the toilet and trying a second time to eliminate more urine. Being pregnant with a baby sitting on the top of the bladder can distort the shape of the bladder and the urethra. ~DBS

Pads

Before you reach your goal, you might need protection. That necessitates using pads. We have been told numerous times that approximately one-third of all feminine hygiene pads sold are actually used for urinary incontinence. Your leak is their lucre.

The problem is that feminine hygiene pads were not designed for incontinence. They are not absorbent enough to keep us dry. Feminine hygiene pads can absorb 100 ml to 350 ml of liquid. Urinary pads can absorb 1000 ml to 2000 ml. What kind of protection do you want?

Specialty pads are designed to form a special gel that holds urine away from the skin. Urine and wetness can be a major irritant where you least want it. These well-designed pads are much thinner than they used to be. Use them. Your skin will remain healthier.

CHAPTER SIX
Biofeedback & Devices

Simple procedures and devices that can be extremely helpful for bladder control:

Biofeedback

Biofeedback may sound very vague and not too scientific. To the contrary, biofeedback is widely used and accepted in clinical medicine. Biofeedback is simply an indicator or measure of a body's function or response that is not otherwise apparent. It is likely that you have one or more biofeedback devices in your home. Taking a person's temperature (thermometer) or blood pressure (blood pressure cuff) requires biofeedback. Standing on the scale for a weight-check is biofeedback. People with diabetes use biofeedback (a glucometer) to test the sugar level of their blood.

Biofeedback for urinary incontinence is available in office, clinical settings or home use. It is safe, effective and can enhance treatment already subscribed such as surgery or medicinal supplements. Generally, biofeedback is managed by a clinician using sensors to relay readings of your muscle contractions to the biofeedback equipment. Pelvic muscle exercises are not difficult, but they can be tricky to execute. The biofeedback tells you and the clinician if you are exercising correctly, how strong your contraction is and how long the contraction lasts. The information retrieved gives you a point of reference in regard to your progress and shows the increased strength and endurance of your pelvic muscles. Immediate and positive reinforcement is key to any successful therapy. Goals become obvious, attainable. This is usually done once a week for four to six office visits.

A portable pelvic-floor muscles trainer called the Myself™ is an over-the-counter device that can provide data similar to biofeedback in the privacy of your own home. Myself™ can be used with each exercise session. The Myself™ unit is like a set of weights in a home gym. You are more likely to do your bicep curls if you have a set of hand weights at home. Similarly, the unit is a convenient and reliable addition to your personal fitness regimen.

Devices

In treating incontinence or pelvic organ prolapse, a health care provider might suggest using one or more of the following devices to augment treatment:

Pessaries

Pelvic support devices, or pessaries, can be inserted into the vagina to provide support for the vaginal walls or uterus. These support devices come in a variety of shapes and sizes, depending upon the patient's needs. They fill space in the vagina that is normally an empty space.

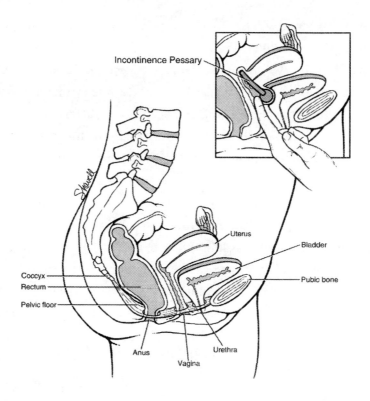

Incontinence Pessary

Uterus

Bladder

Coccyx

Pubic bone

Rectum

Pelvic floor

Anus

Urethra

Vagina

They can provide support to the front of the vagina, back of the vagina, top of the vagina or all three areas. They are fitted by a physician or nurse practitioner. Once properly fitted, the pelvic support device should not be uncomfortable or interfere with urination or bowel movements. The patient is usually unaware of its presence. Some women remove and clean their own device. Others return to their health care provider to have the device removed and cleaned. Either way, the woman using a pelvic support device must have follow-up exams pertaining to proper fit, tissue irritation and effectiveness.

Vaginal Cones or Weights

Vaginal cones are tampon-like devices of increasing weights that are inserted into the vagina. This is resistance training. A woman holds the cone successfully in place for a specified amount of time and then switches to a heavier weight. The ultimate goal is to strengthen the pelvic floor muscles.

The lightest weight cone offers some resistance for the muscle contraction. Over a few days, as her muscle gets stronger, a woman advances to a cone with a greater weight. Next, after strengthening the muscle more, she should try some exertion while the weights are in place, such as coughing or jumping. Think of it as vaginal gymnastics. These cones weigh 20 to 70 grams. While that does not sound heavy, you would not want to drop the heaviest one on your toe. A set of weighted vaginal cones can cost from $135 to $155. They should be made of a safe, smooth, medical grade material and cleaned thoroughly between each use. They should not be shared with anyone else. You should not use them if you have a vaginal infection, irritation, or if they cause discomfort.

Electrical Stimulation—"E-Stim"

E-stim is a process during which an electronic device sends a signal to the pelvic floor muscle to contract. Unlike biofeedback, which records muscle signals, electrical stimulation actually exercises the muscles electronically. This device is often used when there are neurological changes to the bladder or when a patient is having trouble learning how to correctly use her pelvic muscles.

The clinician uses E-stim to help the patient learn the location of the pelvic floor muscles and to get accustomed to the sensation of a contraction. This procedure is performed in an office or clinical setting by a trained health care provider. E-stim might be slightly uncomfortable, but it is not painful. It is most effective when done in conjunction with correct pelvic muscle exercises on a consistent basis.

Electromagnetic Innervation

Electromagnetic innervation is a new technology that uses pulsed magnetic fields to stimulate the nerves and muscles of the pelvic floor to contract. There is no electric current or pain that makes the patient feel uncomfortable. This therapy is available in a clinic or office setting and requires multiple appointments.

CHAPTER SEVEN

Medications, Surgery & Beyond

Medications

Medications are frequently used to treat urge incontinence (UI). Medications designed to inhibit the nerve paths to the bladder can be effective in reducing the activity (or over activity) of the bladder. Although medications can offer relief, taking the right one can be a process of trial and error.

There are many drugs and, unfortunately, they all have side effects. If one drug does not suit you, ask your health care provider about other choices. Extended-release formulas or skin patches may help minimize the number and intensity of side effects.

Think of medication as a first and, sometimes, temporary step in the rehabilitation of your bladder. Your goal is to regain self confidence and control of your life.

Here are some of the most effective therapies available:

1. **Anticholinergics** calm the automatic nerve supply to the bladder to prevent incontinence associated with over active bladder (OAB).

2. **Oxybutynin,** commercially sold as Ditropan™ but also available in a generic formulation, has been available for a long time. It relaxes the smooth muscle of the bladder wall, calming the nerves around it. Ditropan XL™ delivers medication at a steady rate over a 24-hour period. Avoiding the sharp peaks and valleys of treatment with some medications, Oxybutynin also has fewer side effects.

3. **Tolterodine** (sold as Detrol™ in the United States and as Detrusitol™ in Europe) might target the bladder better than other anticholinergics. It offers the advantage of a once-daily dosage and reduces the incidence of one common side effect, dry mouth.

4. **Antidepressants** are sometimes prescribed for the treatment of OAB and SUI. **Imipramine (Tofranil™)** has the advantage of alleviating urge incontinence as well as mild forms of stress incontinence. **Doxepin (Sinequan™)** is appropriate for patients whose bladders are overactive, sensitive and painful as well.

Varying degrees of side effects such as dry mouth, dry eyes, constipation and urine retention (voiding more slowly than normal is usual or not having to urinate at all) have all been associated with the use of drug therapies for OAB. Consult your doctor before taking any medicine.

There is no specific pill that cures stress incontinence without causing other effects. Before taking any medication, discuss your options with your physician or practitioner.

Surgery

Surgery is very often used to treat stress incontinence in women after a variety of behavioral options have failed. There are more than 200 variations of surgical procedures for female stress incontinence, and techniques are being developed all the time to refine practices. You may have heard of some of them: anterior vaginal repair, bladder suspension, sling or specifically named for the physician credited to the procedure. Some very commonly used procedures are the *Marshall/Marchetti/Krantz (MMK)*, *Raz, Stamey,* and the *Burch* procedures. Many of the surgical procedures are designed to add support for the position of the bladder and/or the urethra by tightening or anchoring the connecting tissues. These can correct the angle between the bladder and the urethra (important for continence in the female) and add support for the bladder and urethra. The organs can then work together for bladder control.

New arthroscopic outpatient surgical procedures are available to deal with hyper mobile urethras. The most common procedures in today's market are known as Transvaginal Tape (TVT) or Transobturator Tape (TOT). They are done under local anesthetic and generally do not involve a hospital stay.

Another approach consists of injecting material (such as collagen) around the urethra to add bulk, helping it to close and seal more effectively. Or an artificial sphincter (cuff) or valve might be implanted around the urethra that can be opened and closed as needed to let urine drain.

If you are a stress-incontinence patient, surgery might be the right choice. Discuss this with your physician or practitioner. Be aware of your options and know what you can do to work with your doctor to improve your results, no matter which therapy is used. If you do require surgery, prepare yourself for complete recovery. Do not lift, push or strain with a bowel movement until totally healed. Start Pelvic P yramid exercises when cleared to do so to add support. Behavioral options can always be combined with surgery and medications. Research has shown that pelvic floor exercises increase both the effectiveness of surgery and medications.

When dealing with urgency/frequency, surgery is less common. That is because stress incontinence is frequently related to structural problems and urge incontinence is related to the nerve impulses to the bladder or to something irritating the lining of the bladder. There is, however, a surgical procedure for severe cases of urge incontinence. A device is implanted that provides electrical stimulation to inhibit the sacral nerve and reduce impulses to the bladder. This is known as "neuromodulation," and one of the products on the market is called InterStim™. Neuromodulation is being used by urologists to treat urge incontinence that has not responded to conventional, less invasive, treatments. It is a surgical procedure used in a select population of people suffering with overactive bladder or chronic pelvic pain. There are current trials to assess the use of InterStim™ with patients with multiple sclerosis. If you feel you would be a candidate for any of these procedures, discuss the options with your health care provider.

Real People Update

In the first section of the book, we highlighted some women who had bladder control problems. Before we move on, let us share the rest of their story, their treatment paths.

ANN

Ann's goal was to **decrease the number of day-time leaks** and to **sleep through the night.**

Ann started pelvic muscles exercises with Total Control™. She also reduced her coffee intake and increased her water intake. Eventually Ann learned to perform the "Knack" before she would laugh, cough, sneeze or lift her child. By week four of her exercise program, she was beginning to see progress in her symptoms. By week seven, Ann was sleeping through the night. She no longer feels the need to wear a pad. An occasional 'accident' is now a rare occurrence rather than an everyday incidence.

ANGIE

Angie's goal was to **reduce the number of times that she goes to the bathroom** during the day.

Since behavioral therapy is most often suggested as the first line of defense for treating incontinence, Angie looked at the quality of the liquids she was drinking. She reduced her intake of bladder irritating drinks, coffee and soda, and drank more water. She also practiced pelvic floor exercises and urge suppression by letting her urge pass and waiting 15 minutes before going to the bathroom. Angie started to see improvements within four weeks and was able to wait hours between trips to the bathroom, a major accomplishment for someone who is constantly thinking about the bathroom.

FRAN

The goal for Fran was to **get through the night** without getting her clothing and bed wet.

An assessment and a 24-hour bladder/fluid diary were recorded for Fran. It was discovered that she was drinking several cups of hot chocolate a day with artificial sweetener. She started with a combination of pelvic muscle exercises, a toileting schedule, and fluid management. She practiced urge suppression by taking a deep breath, relaxing, and doing a pelvic muscle contraction, then slowly moving to the bathroom. She reduced her intake of cocoa and artificial sweeteners to one cup a day and increased her water intake. Fran was shown cotton continence underwear with a super absorbent pad insert. With appropriate undergarments, she no longer had to worry about wetting the bed. While this may not be her optimal choice, this was a reasonable choice, realizing how many things she had tried and her desire to get through the night.

CHAPTER EIGHT

Special Topics: Incontinence During Exercise, Pregnancy, Menopause, or Sex

Exercise

Some women experience bladder control problems only when they exercise. This is not uncommon. Up to one-third of women who do vigorous exercise will have some degree of urinary incontinence. It is startling that this has not been addressed, for college athletes, for Olympians, for professional athletes. What secrets we women can keep!

Female athletes generally have well-developed abdominal muscles. However, very few have had training in developing the muscles in their pelvic floor. The bladder and urethra may be in proper position during walking and effortless activities. But some women might leak occasionally while playing tennis or while jumping on the trampoline with the children. Others might experience routine urine leaks while jogging or doing aerobics.

A study of female athletes at a major Midwestern university showed that 28% of the females, average age 19.9 years, had urine loss while participating in their sport. Forty percent of these women first noted urinary leakage problems while in high school, and 17% first noticed problems while in junior high. These women were all elite, physically fit, collegiate athletes who had not experienced pregnancy and childbirth. Their major risk factor for urinary leakage was exercise. Obviously, not everyone who has a bladder control problem is an overweight older mother of several children. The sports associated with the most severe bladder control problems, in descending order, were gymnastics (67%), basketball (66%), tennis (50%), field hockey, track, swimming, volleyball, softball and golf.[8]

THINGS YOU CAN DO

There are several ways to prevent exercise incontinence and the approaches may be combined.

The first is **fitness and/or preventive programs** to develop strength in the pelvic floor muscles, like Total Control™. This can help minimize pelvic floor relaxation and the slight drop of the bladder.

A second approach is the **use of a pelvic floor support device** (pessary) while exercising. This can be as simple as inserting a tampon or pelvic support device in the vagina during exercise, giving enough support to the urethra for complete closure.

A third option is **surgical correction** of pelvic floor relaxation or prolapse. If this is chosen, pelvic floor muscle exercises should be performed after recovery so the muscles can continue to provide support.

Pregnancy and After Childbirth

Women, as child-bearers, have added stress on their pelvic floor that men never experience. That may be why at least two-thirds of all urinary incontinence cases are found in women. One of the most remarkable wonders of the female body is its ability to carry and deliver one newborn infant or more. The fact that a pear-sized organ, the uterus, can expand that much is a physiological feat.

---

8   "Urinary Incontinence in Elite Nulliparous Athletes," Nygaard IE, Thompson FL, Svengalis SL & Albright JP, *Obstetrics and Gynecology*, 1994: 84, pgs 183-187

The tissues of the uterus, the blood vessels, the nerves and the muscles must all stretch to accommodate the bodily changes.

That said, women who have not been pregnant can have incontinence, but risk factors increase with pregnancy. It is the function of the pelvic floor, a structure of muscles and ligaments, to support organs of the pelvis. This includes the uterus, bladder, urethra and rectum. Proper support of these organs is important for eliminating urine. Ligaments attach the muscles to the pelvic bones. Ligaments can stretch to a point, but then they lose elasticity, tear or both. Muscles have more stretch capability than do ligaments. The nerves and blood vessels that run through the pelvic floor also have some stretch capability. During pregnancy, as the baby's weight increases, the pressure on the pelvic floor increases. As the uterus enlarges, the bladder is displaced. A pregnant woman often feels a need to go the bathroom more frequently, because her bladder does not have as much room in the pelvis to expand. She may also leak a little urine when she coughs, laughs, sneezes or lifts an object.

As the baby grows, the pelvic floor must accommodate the weight. If the child is delivered vaginally, rather than by caesarian section, the opening has to stretch wide enough to accommodate the child's head. The bladder, rectum, nerves and blood vessels are compressed against the pelvic bones. A large child, or prolonged labor, can cause the ligaments to tear slightly and nerves to be injured by the stretch. This can lead to a relaxation of the pelvic floor and a loss of support for the bladder, uterus and urethra. The risk of injury increases with each subsequent pregnancy and vaginal delivery.

Many women who have difficulty controlling their bladders during pregnancy recover shortly after delivery. However, with each subsequent pregnancy, recovery may take longer or may not be complete. A young mother may find that she leaks urine when she picks up her 6-month-old child, a symptom of stress incontinence.

Things You Can Do

Following are variables that can affect the status of the pelvic floor after delivery: the difficulty and length of labor, the size and position of the infant or infants, the size of the mother's pelvis, episiotomy, the number of pregnancies and the availability of medical care. Each person and each delivery is unique.

Before Pregnancy

If you have already had your child and are experiencing urinary leakage, prevention is too late for you. But it is not too late to minimize your incontinence risks with subsequent pregnancies. Pelvic muscle exercise in a program like Total Control™ is a technique for strengthening the support of the pelvic floor. Having your pelvic floor muscles and ligaments conditioned and toned is important before getting pregnant. Athletes do not participate in their sport without first getting their leg, back, shoulder and neck muscles conditioned and strong. That would be a foolish risk of injury. Why would a female submit her pelvic floor to the extreme stress of pregnancy and vaginal delivery without being in the best condition?

Exercising the pelvic floor muscles correctly (See Chapter 3) can help reduce stretch injury to the pelvic muscles and incontinence. The exercises must be performed correctly and consistently to get the maximal benefit. Many women believed they were doing Kegels, but because of incorrect contractions were not strengthening their muscles.

Avoid dehydration before, during and after pregnancy. This leads to constipation and straining to have a bowel movement which increases the pressure and forces down the pelvic floor. Eat plenty of fruits, vegetables and fiber, and drink plenty of water during the day. Fluids also keep the urine diluted which is less irritating to the bladder. Avoid coffee, tea, sodas or other agents that can be bladder irritants. For some women, these can cause symptoms of frequency and urgency.

During Pregnancy

Avoid excessive pressure on your pelvic muscles, when possible. This means avoid lifting heavy objects and standing for long periods of time. Rest with your feet elevated when possible. Perform pelvic muscle exercises daily.

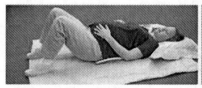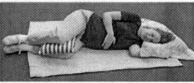

Young pregnant woman doing pelvic muscle exercises. Note positions and use of pillows for comfort.

After Pregnancy

Allow time for your pelvic floor muscles, ligaments, nerves and blood vessels to heal. Do not lift heavy objects, get off your feet when you can, avoid straining with bowel movement and resume your pelvic muscle exercises.

Normally, the pelvic floor contracts by reflex of the nervous system. Immediately after childbirth, this reflex can be lost. If there has been significant pain, trauma, episiotomy, stitches or tearing during delivery, a reflex inhibition can occur. This is nature's way of protecting a swollen, injured or painful area. As healing occurs, teach your pelvic floor muscle to recover its natural reflex action when coughing, sneezing, laughing or lifting. In other words, brace your muscle for the upcoming force.

Many women take a positive approach to returning their bodies to their pre-pregnant state. However, the pelvic floor is unseen and usually forgotten. The pelvic floor can suffer from fatigue as much as any other muscle in the body. A new mother needs rest for recovery.

Do not hesitate to discuss your symptoms with your doctor. It is very common to have urinary incontinence after childbirth. But do not accept it as a lifelong consequence. As soon as you have been cleared by your doctor to exercise, a program such as Total Control™ is a good first step back to health and fitness.

Menopause

It is exciting to discuss the once unmentionable topic of menopause. Two hundred years ago, many women did not live long enough to experience menopause. One hundred years ago, those women who did reach menopause did not talk about it. Today, women are facing the changes that accompany menopause and actively looking for ways to remain in control.

Menopause refers to the cessation of ovarian function (production of estrogen) and menses (monthly period), the end of the reproductive years for a woman. *Note: it refers to the end of REproductive years, not PROductive years.* Today there are approximately 50 million women in the United States who have experienced menopause. Many women today can expect to live one-third of their life after menopause in a very vital manner.

There are several well known health issues related to menopause. They include bone loss (osteoporosis), hot flashes, mood swings, and changes in one's sex life, cardiovascular risks and Alzheimer's disease. Less publicized are the effects of menopause, or loss of estrogen, on a woman's urinary tract and pelvic floor. Urinary incontinence can occur at any age during a woman's life. But many women, up to one-quarter of menopausal women, notice that symptoms begin or seem to worsen around this time.

The vaginal and urinary tissues in a woman are very sensitive to a decreased amount of estrogen. The hormone plays a role in the strength of the pelvic floor muscles and ligaments and in the moisture of the vaginal and urethral tissues. For the urethra to close completely to prevent leakage, it requires a certain degree of elasticity and moisture. Women may experience an increase in stress incontinence and in bladder activity or urge incontinence with menopause. Estrogen also affects the blood flow to the pelvic tissues, causing the lining of the vagina and urethra to be thinner, drier and more easily inflamed. Many women complain of vaginal dryness, itching or irritation with menopause. Vaginal intercourse may become uncomfortable. The urethral tissues may have similar changes and symptoms such as frequency, urgency, urinary tract infections or bladder leakage.

THINGS YOU CAN DO

Menopausal women today are, for the large part, healthy and active. They are concerned about fitness and quality of life. Bladder control and sexuality are priorities. Women are looking to health care practitioners to help provide solutions.

Replacement estrogen can be applied topically to the vagina as a cream or inserted vaginally as a suppository or via a pessary. Locally applied estrogen can help strengthen pelvic floor tissues, improve prolapse and decrease irritable bladder symptoms such as (urgency and frequency). The tissues become thicker and moister. The urethra is able to close tighter, reducing the risk of urinary leakage.

If considering estrogen replacement therapy, discuss all of your options with your health practitioner. This advice applies even if you are considering natural or holistic estrogen sources. Sometimes supplemental estrogen should not be used. Generally, women with breast, uterine or cervical cancer or women with a history of blood clots or stroke are not a candidate for systemic estrogen replacement.

There is no "one answer fits all" in regards to hormone replacement therapy. If you are not able to use estrogen replacement, there are vaginal moisturizers available over the counter. These can provide some relief for vaginal dryness and itching.

Menopause and Your Pelvic Floor

If you are a person who has reached menopause with no thought to your pelvic floor, you need to know that your pelvic floor tissues will only get weaker with age. That means your risks increase for incontinence, prolapse (uterus drops), cystocele (bladder bulges in the vagina) and rectocele (rectum bulges in the vagina). But, it is not too late. You can do a great deal to help yourself.

Strengthening the pelvic floor muscles with exercises and biofeedback, bladder training, weight loss (if needed) and hormone replacement therapy can all help to counter the effects that menopause has on the pelvic floor and bladder tissues. These behavioral therapies can also help to reduce the symptoms of stress and urge incontinence that are associated with menopause.

If you already have prolapse, you may not be able to eliminate it, but you can keep it from becoming worse by strengthening your pelvic floor muscles. Pelvic support devices (pessaries) can also be used to provide support and relieve symptoms of pelvic floor weakness. These devices can often offer sufficient support to decrease urinary incontinence.

Menopause is often a time when women become aggressive about their health. They take supplemental vitamins, exercise, eat healthier, enjoy sexual activity and get screening exams (mammograms). It is a natural time to take a more active role in pelvic floor health and continence.

If you are not yet in the menopause or peri-menopause stage, the message is THE EARLIER, THE BETTER. Start now to get your pelvic floor muscles strong and toned. Be more prepared than your mother was for menopause by doing your pelvic floor muscle exercises correctly and consistently. It is never too late to exercise and increase muscle strength. Practice weight management, adequate fluid intake, and good bladder habits and avoid lifting or exercises that increase pressure on the pelvic floor. **Be Strong, Be Sexy, and Be in Control!**

Sex

Urinary incontinence during sexual activity is a very personal and private issue that is rarely discussed. But, it occurs. It happens mostly in women who have symptoms of stress incontinence, meaning they leak urine with exertion or activity. It can also occur in women with symptoms of urge incontinence. Sexual intercourse can cause urinary leakage from exertion and position changes. Urine can also leak from the bladder as the perineal muscles contract during orgasm or climax. If you or your partner has problems with sexual activity, you can talk to a health care practitioner. Rest assured there are many other couples with this same problem.

Many health issues can affect sexual activity, desire, and one's own image. People with arthritis in their hips or back may find intercourse difficult or certain positions painful. A variety of health problems (diabetes, vascular disease, stroke, depression) and/or medications can affect a woman's ability to experience pleasurable sex. These health problems do not diminish the love between two people. But sexuality is an intimate form of communication and the need for intimacy is greater during illness or chronic health problems. Therefore, it is important to address this situation and search for solutions.

Urine leakage during sexual intercourse can occur during penetration or during orgasm. Incontinence during penetration is likely stress incontinence from the pressure of the penis on the back of the bladder wall or the bladder base. (Remember, the female bladder lies just in front of the vagina.) Usually, the woman would have symptoms of stress incontinence at other times, such as when she laughs or coughs. Strengthening the pelvic floor muscles might help this type of incontinence and even enhance sexual enjoyment for the couple. A small pelvic support device might help, too, and still not interfere with intercourse.

Incontinence during orgasm is likely related to urge incontinence, when the bladder is provoked to instability by the orgasm. It is possible to help this type of incontinence by taking an urge incontinence medication a few hours before planned intercourse.

THINGS YOU CAN DO

Seek help from your doctor and do exercises to strengthen your pelvic muscles. Urinary leakage during sexual activities does not sound very romantic. But urine is sterile when it comes out of the body. It is not dirty. It is cleaner than your mouth (kisses) and probably cleaner than your hands (caresses). A little urine will not hurt your partner. To minimize leakage, go to the toilet before sex play begins. Attempt to double void and empty your bladder. If necessary, place a pad under you on the bed (or wherever) for extra protection. Have a washcloth nearby, "just in case." Know that you are not the only one. Consider the problem of incontinence during sex as unfortunate, but manageable. The emotional expression and closeness of sexual activity are much more important than the physical act.

Communication is so important, yet most of us do not talk about private health issues. Urinary leakage and sex must be the ultimate personal issue. Be brave. Do not suffer with this problem in silence. If you are having incontinence, explain the circumstances to your partner. Ask for understanding and patience. After all, you want the intimacy to continue, too.

After your sex play, take a shower together. Do not make this issue "an end of the world" or tragic scenario. Urinary incontinence affects many people, young and old. Making excuses to avoid sexual activity will only leave your partner wondering if something is wrong. You do not want somebody to feel undesirable or less loved.

Do not let incontinence control your life or interfere with your everyday activities. Continue to exercise, travel, attend social events and have sex. If you are a woman in a warm and loving sexual relationship who "leaks" during intercourse, find solutions together.

If you are the partner of a woman who has incontinence during sexual activity, be supportive. Keep a sense of humor. Help with the hygiene part and carry on with a matter-of-fact and loving attitude. Do not act offended or relate the incontinence to childlike behavior. This analysis could potentially be demeaning or belittling to your partner. As a partner, your acceptance is of great importance. Be tender and touch, so she will not be reluctant to be responsive.

> I had a patient who had stopped sleeping in the same bed with her husband because of her nighttime frequency and sometimes bedwetting. His interpretation was that she did not love him anymore when, in fact, she was doing it out of consideration for him. After he brought up his concerns to me, I guided them towards saying to each other what they had said in private to me. He wanted her closeness and was not willing to lose it because of her incontinence. ~DBS

IN SUMMARY

Congratulations! You are well on your way to enjoying bladder health. Together, we have looked at the basic physiology of the bladder. We have reviewed a variety of medical issues. We have suggested solutions, some that require professional assistance and others that can be tried at home. Perhaps, most importantly, we now know that we are not alone. "You Go Girl!" rings truer everyday. We walk with you on the journey to bladder health and always welcome your feedback and questions. Ours is a passionate partnership. Send us your thoughts, comments and success stories to info@womenshealthfoundation.org

APPENDIX 1:

Self-Discovery

The information in this section will not only help you identify some of your own risk factors for incontinence, but will also quantify the number of leaks and voids per day that you are now having, as well as the severity impact. This will give you a comparison for after you have implemented some behavioral techniques.

Personal Health Background

What are your risk factors? Check the following risk factors that apply to you:

Female

_____ childbirth (how many _____)

_____ hysterectomy

_____ menopause

_____ previous radiation therapy to the pelvis

General

_____ age (over 50)

_____ overweight

_____ smoker

_____ partake in high impact exercises or exertion

_____ high caffeine intake (coffee, tea, soda, chocolate)

Following Conditions

_____ stroke

_____ Parkinson's

_____ diabetes

Are there any of the above risk factors that you can control? Highlight those.

> NOTE: Be sure to share this information with your health care provider for a specific and overall assessment and treatment plan. This does not take the place of an assessment by your health care provider, but is information that can be given to your provider to assist him/her in your diagnosis and treatment plan. This book is designed to provide general information and practical suggestions to help you become a more active participant in dealing with your symptoms. ~DBS

Self Assessment

MEDICAL HISTORY

a) Diabetes, stroke, Parkinson's, arthritis, lower back injury (indicate which)

b) Radiation therapy to pelvic area

c) Birth defect, type _____

MOBILITY

a) Need assistance getting to bathroom (i.e. cane, walker, another person etc.)

b) Need assistance getting clothing up

c) Have fallen within the past year with attempt to get to the bathroom.

Bowel Habits

Frequency
a) Once or more per day

b) Every 2-3 days

c) Every 4 or more days

Characteristics
a) Must strain to have bowel movement

b) Must use assistance to have bowel movement (enema, suppository, laxative)

Urinary Symptoms
a) Blood in urine

b) Pain or burning with urination

c) Strong or foul odor of urine

d) Difficulty in starting to urinate

Frequency of Urine Leaks
a) Once per day

b) 2-3 times per day

c) More than 3 times per day

d) Only at night

e) Number of times to bathroom per night _____

Activities Related to Urine Leaks
a) Coughing, laughing, sneezing, lifting

b) Exercising (jogging, aerobics, etc.)

c) Transferring from chair, getting out of bed, standing

d) On the way to toilet

e) Sexual intercourse

Onset of Urinary Leakage

a) After hysterectomy

b) After childbirth

c) Within past 6 months

d) Within past 2 years

e) Over 2 years

Amount of Urine Leaked

a) A little, minimal

b) A moderate amount

c) A large amount

BLADDER HABITS

Complete with the time you went to the bathroom,
time you leaked, amount and time of fluid intake   Date: _____

Time	Void	Urine Leak Yes/No	Pad Change Yes/No	Fluid Intake*	Comments**
12 a.m.					
1 a.m.					
2 a.m.					
3 a.m.					
4 a.m.					
5 a.m.					
6 a.m.					
7 a.m.					
8 a.m.					
9 a.m.					
10 a.m.					
11 a.m.					
12 p.m.					
1 p.m.					
2 p.m.					
3 p.m.					
4 p.m.					
5 p.m.					
6 p.m.					
7 p.m.					
8 p.m.					
9 p.m.					
10 p.m.					
11 p.m.					
12 p.m.					

*Amount and type (i.e. 1 cup of coffee). **Did you leak a small or large amount, was your pad wet, did you leak on the way to the bathroom or before. What were you doing at the time (sneezing, exercising, having sex, lifting, etc.)

Please complete the 24-hour bladder habit sheet then fill in the following:

1. How many times a day (24-hour) did I leak urine? _____

2. How many times a day did I go to the toilet a day? Add leaks + number of times urinated for total _____

3. How many times did I get up to go to the bathroom at night?

4. What was the average length of time between my voids?

5. How much fluid did I drink, in ounces? 8 oz = 1 cup, 10 oz = 1 glass.

6. Circle any of the following that you may have had in the 24 hours and the amount in ounces or number.

Amount

- Coffee _____
- Cola _____
- Citrus fruit juice _____
- Citrus fruit _____
- Chocolate_____
- Alcohol_____
- Artificial sweetener _____
- Spicy foods _____
- Tomato or tomato juice _____

How Do I Manage My Symptoms?

Pads, tissue, towels, adult diapers, tampon, catheter, devices, scheduled toileting, medications. If you use pads or devices list type and number per day: _____

Skin Care Used for Incontinence

a) Soap

b) Moisturizer

c) Wipes

How do I rate the impact and severity of my symptoms on my life? Complete the stress and urge incontinence severity indices.

Stress Incontinence Severity Index

Circle the appropriate number	Less Than Half the Time	More Than Half the Time
Over the past month how often have you leaked urine while laughing, coughing, lifting, sneezing, having sexual intercourse or exercising?	1	3
Over the past month when you have leaked urine is it a:		
Few drops?	1	3
Moderate Amount?	4	6
Large Amount?	7	9
Does Urinary leakage affect any of the following for you?		
Work?	1	3
Travel?	1	3
Social Activities?	1	3
Exercise?	1	3
Sexual Activity?	1	3

TOTAL POINTS _____

    Symptoms: Mild = 0-10

           Moderate = 11-21

           Severe = 22-27

SELF-RATING SCALE

On a scale of 1 to 10 (with 10 being the worst) how do you rate the severity of your incontinence at this time?

        1 2 3 4 5 6 7 8 9 10

Urge Incontinence Severity Index

Circle the appropriate number	Less Than Half the Time	More Than Half the Time
Over the past month how often have you had the urge to urinate yet leaked urine before reaching the toilet?	1	3
Over the past month how often do you have to get up at night to urinate?		
1 time?	1	3
2-3 times?	4	6
More than 3 times?	7	9
Over the last month have you had to urinate more than once in a two-hour period?	1	3
Does urinary leakage affect any of the following for you?		
Work?	1	3
Travel?	1	3
Social Activities?	1	3
Exercise?	1	3
Sexual Activity?	1	3

TOTAL POINTS _____

    Symptoms: Mild = 0-10

              Moderate = 11-22

              Severe = 23-30

SELF-RATING SCALE

On a scale of 1 to 10 (with 10 being the worst) how do you rate the severity of your incontinence at this time?

        1   2   3   4   5   6   7   8   9   10

Fill in your number for your stress symptom index _____

Fill in your number for your urge symptom index _____

If you have three or more points on the stress incontinence severity index, consider that you have symptoms of stress incontinence. Up to 10 points may be considered mild, up to 21 points may be considered moderate incontinence.

If you have three or more points on the urge incontinence severity index, consider that you have symptoms of urge incontinence. Up to 10 points would be mild, up to 22 would be moderate, and anything over 22 would be severe.

If you have three or more points on the urge scale and on the stress scale, consider that you have symptoms of mixed incontinence. Identify the behavioral treatments that are effective for both stress and urge symptoms.

> These numbers are arbitrary. I personally consider three points on either scale severe, any urinary leakage or frequency is considered severe in my mind. The severity scale is just a point scale so you can keep track of the numbers. The real importance is how bothersome the problem is in your life. ~DBS

APPENDIX 2:

Things I Can Do

Management plans specific for the various types of incontinence symptoms are summarized for a quick referral in the following section. Refer to earlier text for more detailed information.

Stress Symptoms

WHO AM I?
- Women with children
- Women who exercise or do physical labor
- Women after menopause
- Women with a chronic cough
- Women who are overweight
- Women who chronically strain to have a bowel movement

WHAT DO I HAVE?
- Symptoms of urinary leakage with laughing, coughing, sneezing, lifting, exercise, standing

HOW CAN I IMPROVE?
- Keep a 24-hour bladder diary to record when you leak
- Begin a pelvic floor muscle exercise program to work on strength and endurance (Total Control™)
- Use home or office biofeedback
- Practice performing the "Knack" before you laugh, cough or sneeze
- Practice double voiding

- Lose weight if needed
- Stop smoking
- Manage constipation
- If past menopause, consider topical estrogen therapy
- Use a pelvic floor support device if recommended by doctor or practitioner

Urge Symptoms

WHO AM I?
- Women with irritable bladder symptoms
- Women with an overactive bladder
- Women who are pregnant
- Women who are past menopause

WHAT DO I HAVE?
- Symptoms of frequency, urgency
- Have to get to bathroom in a hurry
- May go to toilet 15 to 20 times a day, with minimal leakage of urine
- May leak before getting to toilet
- Get up to go to the bathroom several times a night

HOW DO I IMPROVE?
- Keep a 24-hour bladder and fluid sheet
- Record when you leak in relation to what you drink
- Eliminate bladder irritants
- Drink 6 to 8 glasses of water a day (but not in large amounts at one time)
- Drink fluids throughout the day, rather than in 2 to 3 sittings
- Reduce fluid intake after evening meal
- Get bladder infections (if present) treated
- Practice pelvic muscle exercises (Total Control™)
- Use home or in-office biofeedback

- Practice bladder training using urge suppression
- Stop smoking Provide a safe bathroom environment (lighting, handrails)
- If having problems with mobility, work on gait, balance and leg strength, BE safe
- Wear clothing that is easy to remove quickly

Mixed Symptoms

WHO AM I?

- Women with children
- Women who exercise or do physical labor
- Women after menopause
- Women with irritable bladder symptoms
- Women with overactive bladder

WHAT DO I HAVE?

- Leak urine when cough, laugh, sneeze, exercise, lift, stand
- Have to urinate frequently
- Must reach toilet in a hurry
- Get up at night for the bathroom more than once
- Feel strong, almost painful, urge to void

HOW DO I IMPROVE?

- Keep a 24-hour bladder/fluid diary
- Identify fluids or foods that increase urge
- Avoid fluids or foods that make your bladder more active
- Begin a pelvic floor muscle exercise program (Total Control™)
- Do home or office biofeedback
- Do bladder training with urge suppression to increase bladder capacity
- Drink 6 to 8 glasses of water a day (but not in large amounts at once)

- o Drink fluids in small amounts throughout the day, rather than at two or three sittings
- o Practice pelvic muscle contraction before laugh, cough, sneeze, lift or stand (the "Knack")
- o Double void
- o Lose weight if needed
- o Stop smoking
- o Provide a safe bathroom environment (lighting, handbars)
- o Develop good gait, balance and lower limb strength to prevent falls (be safe)
- o Wear clothing easily removed for toileting

Overflow Symptoms

WHO AM I?
- o Women who have had bladder surgery
- o Women who are pregnant
- o Women with constipation
- o Women with urethral stricture or urethral narrowing
- o Women with spinal cord injury
- o Women with diabetes

WHAT DO I HAVE?
- o Not able to get urine stream started
- o Not able to fully empty bladder
- o Go to the bathroom, void a small amount then have to return again in a few minutes
- o Leak small amounts of urine as bladder overflows

HOW DO I IMPROVE?
- o See your doctor for evaluation
- o Practice double voiding
- o Change positions while urinating ("Rock 'n' Roll")

- Press down on your bladder with your hand while trying to urinate
- Do not wait long periods of time (i.e. over 4 to 5 hours) before trying to urinate in the daytime (you don't want your bladder to overfill or bladder muscle to overstretch).

APPENDIX 3:

Total Control™ History

WHEN MOTHERHOOD CREATES THE NECESSITY FOR INVENTION

Missy Lavender, founder of the Women's Health Foundation, shares her story:

How many of us did our "Kegels" or pelvic floor exercises before, during or after our first pregnancy in our "Preparation for Childbirth" classes? I vaguely remember being talked through an instructive couple of squeezes or two, something about an elevator going up five floors comes to mind. What I can't recall is whether the instructor told me at the time why to do these exercises at this critical juncture in my pelvic health.

No one shared with me the research that regular pelvic floor exercises done during pregnancy have been shown to lead to faster post-partum recovery of muscle strength. I was never "coached" on the where's, why's, or what's of pelvic floor exercises, in spite of the fact that I was a) a regular exerciser, and b) about to undertake what we call 'The Boston Marathon of the Pelvis.' A difficult labor/delivery left me with complete loss of bladder control, I was stunned. After all, I had been in the gym three days a week throughout my entire pregnancy. I had been working out everything, as it turns out, except for the muscles that matter the most: the ones in my pelvic floor.

Eventually, I was directed to a female urogynecologist in Chicago. Dr. Linda Brubaker told me that like many older, first time moms with the big three "don'ts" in delivery (sustained second stage labor, episiotomies and forceps); my pelvic floor was virtually non-functional. She prescribed a continuum of care that included a referral to a pelvic floor physical therapist, Judy Florendo. Under Judy's direction, I learned all about my pelvic floor muscles - where they are, what they do, how critical they are to overall health, bladder function, and even posture. Beginning to regain control over this part of my body, I also began to talk to women of all ages about their pelvic health and share the message of its importance.

An alarming number of my friends, my mother's friends— women of all ages—are like me, mostly ignorant about this part of their bodies. Most of them had had at least one child.

All of them seemed to have some symptom they were dealing with, be it leaking during exercise, feeling like things "were falling out," or battling that "gotta go, gotta go" feeling. I heard over and over, "But isn't that part of being a mom, a woman or of getting older?" In fact, it is estimated that 1 out of 6 adults suffers from incontinence. The unfortunate result for many of these women was a decrease in their activity level. Former runners were now walkers and former kick boxers were in water aerobic classes. Most women were not doing anything at all for their health and fitness. I began to wonder if there wasn't something missing. Where was the fitness solution for women who leaked? Could we develop something that allowed women with incontinence a "safe" way to move, as well as something that might actually improve their symptoms?

The Total Control™: A Pelvic Wellness Program for Women began in 2004 at the same time that I founded the Women's Health Foundation. An innovative fitness and educational program for women suffering incontinence or other pelvic floor dysfunctions, Total Control™, participants learn a full-body workout centered on the muscles of the Pelvic Pyramid. Created by Canadian physiotherapist, Diane Lee, the Pelvic Pyramid (pelvic floor, the "base", multifidus, the "back", and transversus abdominus or "TVA", the "front") is essential for optimal mobility and stability of all women's bodies.

In the fall of 2004, a pilot research study conducted by Dr. Linda Brubaker at Loyola Medical Center in Chicago found that the program significantly improved or alleviated symptoms of both stress incontinence and urgency/frequency incontinence. We also saw dramatic improvements reported in quality of life. A second clinical research study is currently testing the impact of Total Control™ on everything from overactive bladder symptoms, to sexual health and function.

One of our mantras at Women's Health Foundation is "**Knowledge is Power, Power is Control!**" The other is, "**You Go, Girl, But Only When You Want!**" We believe in the power of the Pelvic Pyramid to change the lives of women who struggle to move and be active in the face of bladder control problems. We look forward to transforming the lives of women everywhere as they, too, take control!

Success Stories

WHO'S THAT MIDDLE-AGED LADY IN PULL-UPS? OR WHY I SIGNED UP TO TAKE THIS CLASS

The following true story will give you an idea why I signed up to take the Total Control™ class.

One winter day, several years ago my family decided to take an outing to the Chinese New Year in China Town. Knowing it would be mobbed, we took a packed El to China Town.

We took our place in the back of what turned out to be throngs of tourists. They were doing the same thing we were, admiring the dragons on a frosty winter day. I stood on a brick or a rock or something so I could get a peek at the parade. I don't know if I tripped or giggled or what. Something jiggled my body. Next thing you know I had pee streaming down my legs. Out of the clear blue in the midst of down town China Town on a frosty winter day.

There was no car to flee to. Struck with the sheer out-of-controllness of the situation, I started to laugh. I crossed my legs and cracked up. I don't need to tell you what happened as I laughed harder and harder.

I experienced a true spiritual surrender. There was absolutely nothing I could do. It was kind of the ultimate urinary incontinence hitting bottom experience. I was still in a state of denial in those days so I wore no pads or panty liners. Just cotton panties.

Amidst the exotic sights, sounds and smells of China town, there I stood with soaked panties and by now a frosty bottom and legs. With some difficulty, we fought the mobs and found an upstairs bath room in a restaurant where I could clean up a bit. Even my shoes were soaked.

I don't remember if I deep-sixed my panties or not. If I had an ounce of sense I would have. No, come to think of it I did not. I'm having a flash back now, I believe I wadded my underpants with toilet paper and felt extremely grateful to do so.

Believe it or not fellow incontinence sufferers, I did not demand to take the next train home. I sat there with soggy under-wear and who knows what else, and enjoyed the outing with my family. I experienced the true freedom of realizing how little in life we actually have control over and gratitude for the small things in life like a seat in a Chinese restaurant and dry toilet paper.

So, that's the before story. Flash forward to the present. I had been kvetching to my also middle-aged friend, Kathy, about the magnitude of, shall we say, my problem. I thought I was destined to spend my old age in Chucks.

I am a believer in Divine Providence. Kathy heard about this class and neither of us hesitated for a nanno-second to sign up. Here comes the testimonial part.

Do the words, "Dry panties," mean anything to you? After 11 weeks in this course, I am truly symptomatically improved. Shall I pick a number? Probably 80% better on my good days and 60 or so when I fall of the wagon and imbibe in a cup of tea.

The basic Incontinence Education 101 has helped. I used to drink lots of black and green tea. Isn't it amazing how ignorant an otherwise educated health care consumer can be?

The pelvic strengthening has been a real experience, as well. My TVA is on now, whenever I think of it, and taut as a sheet on a bed in military school. I have a new found power as I elevate my pelvic floor and squeeze then relax. Hey, I can do it during meetings.

I have yet to experience the multifidus, but I have a high level of confidence that it does exist and that I will some day. I'm signing up for the advanced course.

The camaraderie and the good will of the instructors and participants have been great. Having other people interested and with you on the journey is a huge piece of the success of the experience. I would never in a million years lie on the floor for two and a half hours a week and squeeze parts that I can not see and I did not even know that I had. I have the attention span of a flea. Left to my own devices without the group support, I shudder to think of what my fate would be.

So, in all seriousness, it's been a great class that was run with a lot of thought and planning. Thanks for all the effort and thought and unabashed enthusiasm that has gone into this experience.

Linda, 48

I can honestly say that since I started the class 4 weeks ago...I haven't had any leakage at all. For me....it would just catch me off guard, like if I sneezed or sneezed the 2nd time. It was never the 1st time, always the 2nd time; I could never control what happened with that and I haven't had any leakage at all since I started the class. So, it makes me feel more confident I can do some active things, some I quit doing, because I had those problems.

Sandy, 42

I've noticed a number of really good things. Number 1, I don't need to go to the bathroom when I go shopping; I can wait till I get home. Number 2, when I cough or sneeze, I can catch it before I leak. Number 3, even when I drink ice tea before bedtime, I can sleep through the night; I don't have to get up at 5:30 and go to the bathroom. I stand taller and straighter; my shoulders are squarer; it's easier to get off the floor.

I think it's one of the best things I've done in years."

Catherine, 75

The changes that I noticed after taking Total Control™ were unexpected. I took Total Control™ because I wanted the information, not because I felt like I had any kind of issue. But what I was surprised to notice was that I could sleep through the night, I didn't wake up in the middle of the night to go to the bathroom; I was able to sleep all night long. It may seem like a simple thing, but when you don't interrupt your night's sleep and you get a full 71/2 or 8 hours, it makes a difference.

Jeanette, 55

Bottom line, it's given me back the quality of life I was missing!

Fran, 85

APPENDIX 4:
References and Resources

Recommended Reading

7 Steps to Normal Bladder Control, E. Vierck. Harbor Press, Inc., Gig Harbor, WA 1998

Atlas of Human Anatomy, Frank H. Netter, M.D. CIBA-GEIGY Corporation, West, Caldwell, NJ, 1989

Conquering Incontinence: A New and Physical Approach to a Freer Lifestyle, P. Dornan. Allen & Unwin, 2003

Beyond Kegels, Second Edition, J.A. Hulme. Phoenix Publishing Company, Missoula, MT, 2002

Bounce Back Into Shape After Baby, Caroline Creager, Berthoud, CO, 2001

Ever Since I Had My Baby, R. Goldberg. Three Rivers Press, New York, 2003

The Female Pelvis: Anatomy & Exercises, B. Calais-Germain. Eastland Press, Seattle, 2003

Female Urology, Urogynecology, and Voiding Dysfunction, S. P. Vasavanda, M.D., et. al. Marcel Dekker, New York, 2005

Fitness for the Pelvic Floor, Beate Carrière, PT. Thieme, New York, 2002

For Women Only: A Revolutionary Guide to Reclaiming Your Sex Life, J. Berman, M.D., and L. Berman, Ph.D. Henry Holt, New York, 2001

Human Sexual Response, W.H. Masters and V.E.Johnson. Little, Brown, Boston, 1966

I Laughed So Hard I Peed My Pants: A Woman's Essential Guide for Improved Bladder Control, K. Berzuk. IPPC, 2002

"Incontinence: New Ways to Stay Dry," *Health.* Better Homes and Gardens. 13 Sept. 2004

The Incontinence Solution: Answers for Women of All Ages, W. H. Parker, et. al. Fireside, New York, 2002

Male and Female Sexual Dysfunction, A.D. Seftel, M.D., editor. Mosby, New York, 2004

Managing and Treating Urinary Incontinence, Diane Kaschak Newman. Health Professions Press, MD, 2002

Mayo Clinic on Managing Incontinence, P. Pettit, editor. Mayo Clinic, Rochester, NY, 2005

"Mind Over Bladder," *Health.* Wendy Lichtman. April 2004: 42-46

Moving Through Menopause, Kathy Smith. Kathy Smith Enterprises, Inc., NY, 2002

"Nonsurgical Treatments for Stress Urinary Incontinence in Women," *Virtual Hospital.* Ingrid Nygaard, M.D., Fall 2001/Feb. 2003. University of Iowa, 19 Oct. 2004

Overcoming Bladder Disorders, R. Chalker and K.E. Whitmore, M.D. Harper Perennial, New York, 1991

Overcoming Incontinence, Mary Dierich, M.S.N., R.N., C.N.P., and Felecia Froe, M.D. Three Rivers Press, 2003

Overcoming Overactive Bladder: Your Complete Self-Care Guide, D.K. Newman and A.J. Wein, M.D. New Harbinger Publications, Oakland, CA, 2004

"Pelvic Exercises for Incontinence in New Moms," *WebMD Health.* Miranda Hitti, 21 Sept. 2004. 11 Oct. 2004

The Pelvic Floor: Its Function and Disorders, Henry, Swash, and John Pemberton. Saunders, May Clinic and Foundation, Rochester, MN, 2001

Pelvic Floor Disorders, Alain Bourcier. Saunders, London, 2004

Pelvic Floor Re-education: Principles and Practice, B. Schüssler, et.al. Springer-Verlag, London, 1994

The Pelvic Girdle 2ⁿᵈ Edition, Diane Lee. Churchill Livingstone, United Kingdom, 1999

Pelvic Health & Childbirth: What Every Woman Needs to Know, M. Murphy, M.D., and C.L. Wasson. Prometheus Books, Amherst, NY, 2003

Pelvic Power for Men and Women: Mind/Body Exercises for Strength, Flexibility,

Posture, and Balance, Eric Franklin. Princeton Book Company, Publishers, Highstown, NJ, 2003

"Pilates Q&A-On the Right Track with the Pelvic Floor," *Pilates Style.* Marie-Jose Blow-Lawrence. Fall 2004: 94

Saving the Whole Woman: Natural Alternatives to Surgery for Pelvic Organ Prolapse and Urinary Incontinence, A.K. Kent. Bridgeworks, Albuquerque, NM, 2003

Secrets of the Sexually Satisfied Woman: Ten Keys to Unlocking Ultimate Pleasure, L. Berman, Ph.D., and J. Berman, M.D., Hyperion, New York, 2005

Sexual Behavior in the Human Female, Kinsey, A.C., et.al. Indiana University Press, Bloomington, Reprint Edition, 1998

Spinal Stabilization-The New Science of Back Pain, 2ⁿᵈ Edition. Rick Jemmet BSc (PT), Novent Health Publishing, Canada, 2003

"Tackling the Teaser," *Pilates Style*. Polly Morrow. Fall 2004: 64

Therapeutic Management of Incontinence and Pelvic Pain. J. Haslam and Laucock (Eds). United Kingdom: Churchill Livingstone, 1999

The Urinary Incontinence Sourcebook, Diane Kaschak Newman, Lowell House, IL NTC/Contemporary Publishing Group, Inc., Los Angeles, 1997, 1999

The V Book: A Doctor's Guide to Complete Vulvovaginal Health, Elizabeth Gunther Stewart, M.D., and Paula Spencer. Bantam Books, New York, 2002

Vaginas: An Owner's Manual, Carol Livoti, M.D., and Elizabeth Topp. Thunder's Mouth Press, New York, 2004

Women's Waterworks: Curing Incontinence, P. Chiarelli. George Perry, 2002

Your Personal Guide to Bladder Health, National Association for Continence, 2001

Online Resources

Agency for Healthcare Research and Quality
www.ahrq.gov

American Academy of Family Physicians
www.familydoctor.org

American College of Obstetricians and Gynecologists
www.acog.org

American Medical Association
www.ama-assn.org

American Medical Women's Association
www.amwa-doc.org

American Physical Therapy Association
www.apta.org

American Urogynecologic Society (AUGS)
www.augs.org

American Urological Association (AUA)
www.urologyhealth.org
www.auanet.org

AUA Foundation, Inc.
www.afud.org

Canadian Continence Foundation
www.continence-fdn.ca

Center for Disease Control and Prevention
www.cdc.gov

Center for Science in the Public Interest
www.cspinet.org

Herman & Wallace, Inc.
Pelvic Rehabilitation Institute
www.pelvicrehab.com

InContiNet
www.incontinet.com

Institute of Medicine of the National Academics
www.iom.edu

International Continence Society (ICS)
www.continet.org

iVillage (Women's Health and Well-Being)
www.ivillage.com

Medicare and Medicaid
www.cms.hhs.gov

Medline Plus®
U.S. National Library of Medicine
National Institutes of Health
www.nlm.nih.gov/medlineplus

National Association for Continence
www.nafc.org

National Enuresis Society
www.peds.umn.edu/center/nes

National Institutes of Health
www.health.nih.gov

National Institute on Aging, NIH
www.nia.nih.gov

National Kidney and Urologic Disease Information
www.kidney.niddk.nih.gov

National Women's Health Resource Center
www.healthywomen.org

RealAge
www.realage.com

The Simon Foundation for Continence
www.simonfoundation.org

Society for Urodynamics & Female Urology
www.sufuorg.com

Society of Urological Nurses and Associates
www.suna.org

U.S. Department of Health and Human Services
www.os.dhhs.gov

U.S. Food and Drug Administration (FDA)
www.fda.gov

The Whole Woman (prolapse information)
www.wholewoman.com

WebMD
www.webmd.com

Women's Health Foundation
www.womenshealthfoundation.org

Women's Sexual Wellness
Association of Reproductive Health Professionals and National Women's
Health Resource Center
www.nutureyournature.org

Pharmaceuticals and Medical Devices

Aris™ T.O.T. (Surgical Sling)
Mentor Corporation
www.mentorcorporation.com

Ditropan® XL (oxybutynin chloride)
Ortho-NcNeil Pharmaceutical, Inc.
www.ditropan.com

Detrol®LA (tolterodine tartrate)
Pfizer, Inc.
www.bladderinfo.com
www.detrolla.com

Enablex® (darifenacin)
Novartis
www.enablex.com

Estrace® (estradiol vaginal cream)
Warner Chilcott PLC
www.estrace.com

Gynecare (Surgical Slings)
Prolift (Prolapse Repair)
Ethicon, Inc. (Johnson & Johnson)
www.gynecare.com

Lynx®, Obtryx® (Surgical Slings)
Coaptite® (Injectable Bulking Agent)
Boston Scientific
www.bostonscientific.com

Medtronic/InterStim® Therapy (Neuromodulation Implant)
www.medtronic.com

Oxytrol® (oxybutynin transdermal system)
Watson Pharma, Inc.
www.bladdercontrol.com
www.oxytrol.com

Premarin® (conjugated estrogens - hormonal vaginal cream)
Wyeth Pharmaceuticals, Inc.
www.premarin.com

Renessa® System (non-surgical SUI treatment)
Novasys Medical, Inc
www.novasysmedical.com

SANCTURA® (trospium chloride)
Esprit Pharmaceuticals, Inc.
Indevus Pharmaceuticals, Inc.
www.sanctura.com

SPARC™, Monarc™, BioArc™ (Surgical Slings)

Perigree®, Apogee® (Prolapse Repair)

AUS (Artificial Urinary Sphincter)

American Medical System (AMS)

www.americanmedicalsystem.com

Uretex®, Uretex®TO (Surgical Slings)

Contingen®, Tegress® (Injectible Bulking Agents)

C.R.Bard, Inc

www.bard.com

Vagifem® (estradiol vaginal tablets)

Novo Nordisk, Inc.

www.vagifem.com

VESIcare® (solifenacin succinate)

Astellas Pharma Inc.

The GlaxoSmithKline Group of Companies

Glossary

Alzheimer disease: A type of dementia, characterized by confusion, memory loss, disorientation.

Bedwetter: Incontinent of urine at night while in bed.

Biofeedback: A process providing a person information about her body through the use of instrumentation, such as blood pressure or muscle contraction.

Bladder: The muscular sac in the pelvis that stores urine.

Bladder control: Ability to voluntarily keep urine from leaking out of the bladder.

Bladder drill: (see bladder training) A system of therapy for incontinence in which a patient practices holding urine for increasing increments of time.

Bladder suspension: A surgical procedure to position the bladder and prevent descent in to the vagina.

Bladder training: Another term for bladder drill, a system of therapy for incontinence in which a patient practices holding urine for increasing increments of time.

Burch procedure: A surgical procedure for stress incontinence, the urethra is stabilized to prevent mobility and leakage.

Chronic incontinence: Urinary leakage that has occurred for over 6 months and not of a temporary nature.

Congestive heart failure: A condition where the heart as a pump cannot perform its functions good enough to keep blood circulating throughout the body.

Constipation: Difficulty in passing stool or passing of hard stools.

Cystocele: Protrusion or hernia of the bladder in to the vagina.

Diabetes: A clinical condition where there is a decrease or lack of insulin secretion to metabolize sugars, characterized by increase in urine output.

Diuretic medication: A drug that promotes the excretion of urine.

Double void: A technique for emptying the bladder, essentially trying to empty the bladder twice in a short space of time.

Elasticity: Ability of tissue to regain its original shape after stretching.

Electrical stimulation: A process where electrodes, either implanted or on the surface of the body, convey a small electrical current for therapeutic purposes.

Estrogen: The female hormone, responsible for secondary sex characteristics of the female, important in vaginal, urethral and pelvic muscle strength.

Multifidus: A very deep back muscle located right next to the bones in the midline of your spine and pelvis. It is a key stabilizer of the back and pelvis which allows your lower back to work effectively and without pain. It also serves as the back of the Pelvic Pyramid.

Neutral Spine: The position of the spine where the load of the trunk is evenly distributed between the anterior and posterior structures of the spinal column. The ideal position for optimal muscle recruitment of TVA and multifidus.

Pelvic Floor Muscles ("PFM"): The pelvic floor consists of a hammock of muscles that connect the pubis at the front to the tailbone (coccyx) and "sitz" or ischial tuberosities at the back. There are three main muscles that make up the pelvic floor - pubococcygeus, iliococcygeus and ischiococcygeus. A woman's urethra, vagina and anus pass through these muscles and are affected by their function. It also serves as the floor or bottom of the Pelvic Pyramid.

Pelvic Pyramid: The transversus abdominus, multifidus and pelvic floor form the Pelvic Pyramid (think "front, back, floor"). The Pelvic Pyramid functions to stabilize and support the pelvis and the spine. It also facilitates proper organ function. Weakness or the inability to recruit any of the Pelvic Pyramid muscles affects the effectiveness of the pyramid as a whole

Rectocele: A protrusion or hernia of the rectum in to the vagina.

Rectum: The portion of the colon just above the anus, or outside opening.

Reflex incontinence: Loss of bladder control related to a problem in the spinal cord.

Self-dehydration: Limiting fluid intake, enough to cause dehydration or excessive loss of water from the body.

Skin breakdown: A break in the skin integrity, an ulcer or abrasion.

Sphincter: A circular band of muscle fibers that can close a natural opening in the bladder, a valve, like the bladder sphincters.

Stress incontinence: Loss of urine related to physical exertion, usually associated with pelvic floor weakness or sphincter insufficiency.

Transient incontinence: Loss of bladder control that is temporary, such as related to a urinary tract infection (treat the infection and the incontinence is resolved).

Transversus Abdominus ("TVA"): The deepest muscle of the four abdominal muscles. It is built like a corset around the trunk and is the only abdominal muscle that attaches to our spinal joints. One function is to stiffen the spine and stabilize the pelvis prior to movements of the arms and legs. It also serves as the front of the Pelvic Pyramid.

Ureters: Two tubes connecting the kidneys to the bladder.

Urethra: Tube connecting the bladder to the outside of the body.

Urge incontinence: Loss of bladder control characterized by frequent and urgent need to go to the bathroom.

Urinary tract infection: Infection of the kidneys or bladder.

Uterus: Female organ of reproduction, lies behind and just above the bladder.

Vagina: Female canal to the uterus, lies behind the bladder and in front of the rectum.

Vaginal weights: Cones designed to be used by females when strengthening the pelvic muscles to treat incontinence.

Voiding: The act of urinating, to empty the bladder.

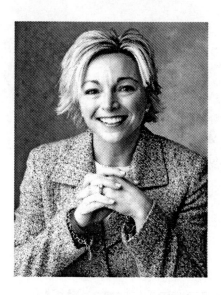

A Letter From Missy Lavender

Eight years ago, I was fit, 40 and about to deliver my first child. I had a model pregnancy, however after undergoing a difficult delivery, I found myself with absolutely no control over my bladder. For six weeks following, I battled the depression and embarrassment of constantly wearing huge pads, not being able to even briskly walk without leaking urine. When I confided this to my OBGYN, she dismissed me, saying, "Go home, do your Kegels and give it six months. You'll be fine."

Four months later, still leaking, I was so depressed I called my psychiatrist friend, begging her for Prozac. This is where I got lucky: instead of the millions of women who suffer in silence, my friend recommended I see a local urogynecologist.

Many times, when we bring this problem up to our doctor, we hear, "This is part of being a mom, getting older, being female." We hear that and we retreat in silence. But this urogynecologist told me I resembled half of her patients—older, first time moms with long 2nd stage labors, episiotomies and forceps deliveries. She also reassured me that telling *me* to go home and "Kegel" was like telling an athlete with a torn muscle to go to the gym and "work it out".

Thankfully, my story has a happy ending. Through physical therapy, exercise and surgery, I am better. However, while going through this life-altering process, I discovered my life's work. The Women's Health Foundation was formed in 2004 with a mission to improve the pelvic health and fitness of women through education, research and innovative programs. We created a fitness and educational program, Total Control™, to work a women's body "from the inside out" by activating three key core muscle groups that affect continence, alignment, sexual pleasure and posture. Women in the class also learn key behavioral tips that can immediately change their bladder and pelvic health.

The first Total Control class launched that same year. Now we train instructors to teach this program in local gyms, YMCA's and hospitals. Classes are running in Denver, Boston, Chicago and recently Anchorage! Our goal is to put pelvic fitness on the map for all women - not just those who leak. Our graduates are fit, knowledgeable about their bodies feel sexier, are more empowered and are certainly, in more control. We call them "Pelvic Floor Evangelists" because they leave us and go out in the world sharing what they know with their girlfriends, sisters and daughters.

My journey to health and fitness has changed my life for the better, but my work with WHF has been a joyful path to help thousands of women reconnect to their true "core", from the inside out!

Missy Lavender, MBA, is the Founder and Executive Director of the Women's Health Foundation in Chicago, Illinois. She received her MBA from the J.L. Kellogg Graduate School of Management at Northwestern University and her B.A. from Miami of Ohio. Ms. Lavender is a national inspirational speaker and has been featured in such publications as *Better Homes & Gardens, Northshore Magazine, The Daily Herald* and *Lifetime in Health.* Ms. Lavender was featured on WGN Channel 9 News and on the PBS show, Real Savvy Moms. She and her family live in downtown Chicago with their dog, Beeb.

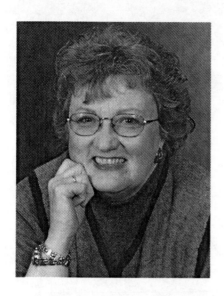

Dorothy B. Smith, R.N., MS, is a nurse who has worked with incontinence patients in acute care and long-term care settings, assisted living, clinics, and home care. She is the author of over 125 professional publications related to her field and has given numerous presentations in the US, Canada, and Europe. She has been editor of The Journal of Wound, Ostomy and Continence Nursing and Dimensions in Oncology Nursing. Ms. Smith has received nursing and publication honors from The University of Texas M.D. Anderson Cancer Center (Brown Award), The Oncology Nursing Society (Mara Mogensen Flaherty Award), the Wound, Ostomy and Continence Nurses Society (manuscript award), The Texas Medical Center (essay award), The American Medical Writers Association (book award) and is a Fellow in The American Academy of Nursing. She is certified by the Wound, Ostomy and Continence Nursing Society. Currently she is Vice President, Clinical Affairs for DesChutes Medical Products, Inc., Bend, Oregon, a research and development company for pelvic floor dysfunction. Dorothy is married and has one daughter.

About the Women's Health Foundation

The Women's Health Foundation, a 501c3 non-profit organization, was formed in 2004 with goal to improve the pelvic health and fitness of all women. Through educational initiatives, programs, and products like this book—we seek to enable women to free themselves and regain total control of their bodies and lives.

As a nonprofit foundation, we rely on your support to fund our organization and research. Please consider us in your giving this year. By giving what you can, our unique foundation will continue to grow and change the lives of women everywhere.

Women's Health Foundation is Paypal™ verified and can accept donations on our website at www.womenshealthfoundation.org. Monetary gifts of any amount can be given in cash, or by check, money order, and credit card. Alternatively, we also accept appreciated securities.

Please send your gift to:
The Women's Health Foundation
632 W. Deming Place
Chicago, IL 60614-2676

If you would like to purchase the Total Control™ Program at-home fitness DVD, *"Be Fit, Be Sexy, Be in Control,"* and/or any other supplementary fitness equipment, go to www.totalcontrolprogram.com.

If you have any questions, contact Molly Kirk, Operations Director, at Women's Health Foundation. Phone: 773-305-8201, Email: molly@womenshealthfoundation.org

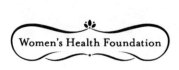

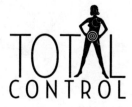

Women's Health Edu. - Chicago integrated program to empower your women

Becky Keller + Juliette Perot — Nurse from virginia
Pelvic Floor P.T

multifidus
Deep back muscles

Pelvic Pyramid

Pelvic floor

Transverse abdominal

CPSIA information can be obtained
at www.ICGtesting.com
Printed in the USA
FFOW05n1810100315

9 780979 687600